This report contains the coll......i...s of an international group of experts and
does not necessarily represent the decisions or the stated policy of the World Health Organization

WHO Technical Report Series
905

CONTROL OF CHAGAS DISEASE

Second report of the
WHO Expert Committee

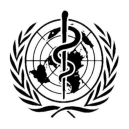

World Health Organization
Geneva 2002

WHO Library Cataloguing-in-Publication Data

WHO Expert Committee on the Control of Chagas Disease (2000 : Brasilia, Brazil)
  Control of Chagas disease : second report of the WHO expert committee.

  (WHO technical report series ; 905)

  1.Chagas disease — prevention and control   2.Chagas disease — transmission
  3.Trypanosoma cruzi   4.Disease vectors   5.Guidelines   I.Title   II.Series

  ISBN 92 4 120905 4   (NLM classification : WC 705)
  ISSN 0512-3054

The World Health Organization welcomes requests for permission to reproduce or translate its publications, in part or in full. Applications and enquiries should be addressed to the Office of Publications, World Health Organization, Geneva, Switzerland, which will be glad to provide the latest information on any changes made to the text, plans for new editions, and reprints and translations already available.

The designations employed and the presentation of the material in this publication do not imply the expression of any opinion whatsoever on the part of the Secretariat of the World Health Organization concerning the legal status of any country, territory, city or area or of its authorities, or concerning the delimitation of its frontiers or boundaries.

The mention of specific companies or of certain manufacturers' products does not imply that they are endorsed or recommended by the World Health Organization in preference to others of a similar nature that are not mentioned. Errors and omissions excepted, the names of proprietary products are distinguished by initial capital letters.

Typeset in Hong Kong
Printed in Singapore
2001/13948 — SNPBest-set/SNPSprint — 7500

Contents

WHO Expert Committee on the Control of Chagas Disease

Brasilia, 20–28 November 2000

Members

Dr J.R. Coura, Director, Oswaldo Cruz Institute (FIOCRUZ), Rio de Janeiro, Brazil (*Chairman*)

Dr J.C.P. Dias, René Rachou Research Centre, Belo Horizonte, Brazil

Dr A.C.C. Frasch, Institute for Biotechnological Research, San Martin National University, Buenos Aires, Argentina

Dr F. Guhl, Director, Centre for Research on Tropical Microbiology and Parasitology (CIMPAT), University of the Andes, Santafé de Bogotá, Colombia (*Rapporteur*)

Dr J.O. Lazzari, Chief, Department of Cardiology, Pirovano Hospital, Buenos Aires, Argentina

Dr M. Lorca, Faculty of Medicine, University of Chile, Santiago, Chile

Dr C. Monroy Escobar, School of Biology, San Carlos University, Guatemala City, Guatemala

Dr C. Ponce, Director, Central Laboratory, Ministry of Health, Tegucigalpa, Honduras

Dr A.C. Silveira, formerly Director, Chagas disease control programme of Brazil, Brasilia, Brazil

Dr G. Velazquez, Institute for Research in the Health Sciences, Asunción, Paraguay

Dr B. Zingales, Biochemical Institute, University of São Paulo, São Paulo, Brazil

Secretariat

Dr J. Finkelman, Country Representative, WHO Regional Office for the Americas/Pan American Sanitary Bureau, Brasilia, Brazil

Dr A. Luquetti, Director, Serodiagnostic Laboratory for Chagas Disease, Federal University of Goias, Goiana, Brazil (*Temporary Adviser*)

Dr A. Moncayo, Manager, Task Force on Chagas Disease, UNDP/World Bank/ WHO Special Programme for Research and Training in Tropical Diseases, WHO, Geneva, Switzerland (*Secretary*)

Dr G. Schmunis, formerly Coordinator, Programme of Communicable Diseases, WHO Regional Office for the Americas/Pan American Sanitary Bureau, Washington, DC, USA (*Temporary Adviser*)

Dr A. Valencia, WHO Regional Office for the Americas/Pan American Sanitary Bureau, Washington, DC, USA

1. Introduction

A WHO Expert Committee on the Control of Chagas Disease met in Brasilia from 20 to 28 November 2000. Dr J. Finkelman, WHO/PAHO Representative in Brazil, opened the meeting on behalf of the Director-General.

Chagas disease occurs throughout Latin America but the disease manifestations and epidemiological characteristics vary from one endemic area to another, and prevalence rates, parasite characteristics, clinical pathology, vectors, and reservoir hosts differ widely. More than any other parasitic disease, Chagas disease is closely related to social and economic development.

Efforts to interrupt the transmission of Chagas disease have been successful in several countries and must continue: cost-effective methods of chemical control of the vectors and blood-bank screening are available. Transmission by blood transfusion has increasingly been reported as the cause of new infections outside the foci of natural transmission.

In the countries of the Southern Cone Initiative (see section 8.1), transmission of Chagas disease was interrupted in Uruguay in 1997, in Chile in 1999, in 8 of the 12 endemic states of Brazil, and in 4 of the 16 endemic provinces of Argentina in 2000. Available data on trends towards reduced infection rates in younger age groups and increased screening of blood banks indicate that transmission (by vector and by transfusion) will be interrupted in the remaining countries, namely Bolivia and Paraguay, by 2003. Interrupting the transmission of Chagas disease in these six countries will substantially reduce the incidence of Chagas disease in the whole of Latin America.

In the light of the progress made by 1998 in the countries of the Southern Cone Initiative, the World Health Assembly, in resolution WHA.51.14, adopted on 16 May 1998, acknowledged the decision of the Andean countries (Colombia, Ecuador, Peru, and Venezuela) and the Central American countries (Belize, Costa Rica, El Salvador, Guatemala, Honduras, Nicaragua, and Panama) to launch similar initiatives (see also p. 87, and sections 8.2 and 8.3, respectively).

In these countries, 5–6 million individuals are infected and 25 million are at risk of contracting the infection. However, as the vectors of Chagas disease concerned are not strictly domiciliated but can reinfest dwellings from sylvatic ecotopes, it will be necessary to develop control strategies appropriate to the local entomological conditions.

In the past decade, most endemic countries have initiated or strengthened national control programmes with remarkable success, as in the Southern Cone Initiative. These programmes have shown that current control methods, if sustained, can be effective. The investments made in terms of national skills, health facilities, and finance reflect a political and technical commitment at national level that is crucial to the development of sustained control programmes.

This report on the second meeting of the WHO Expert Committee on Control of Chagas Disease provides technical guidelines on the planning, implementation, and evaluation of national control programmes to achieve the goal of interruption of transmission. Current knowledge of the disease and its pathogenesis, the parasites and criteria for their classification, and the vectors and reservoirs of infection are critically reviewed. Strategies for the interruption of transmission and their cost-effectiveness are also discussed.

2. Basic information on Chagas disease

2.1 Clinical forms

Chagas disease passes through two successive stages — an acute phase and a chronic phase. The acute phase lasts 6–8 weeks. Once this subsides, most infected patients appear healthy, and no evidence of organ damage can be found by the current standard methods of clinical diagnosis. The infection can be detected only by serological or parasitological tests. This form of the chronic phase of Chagas disease is called the indeterminate form, and in most patients persists indefinitely. However, several years after the chronic phase has started, 10–40% of infected individuals, depending on the geographical area, will develop lesions of various organs, mainly the heart and the digestive system. This condition is called the cardiac or digestive form of chronic Chagas disease. The chronic phase lasts for the rest of the life of the infected individual (*1*).

2.1.1 *Acute phase*

Acute Chagas disease can occur at any age. However, the majority of cases are detected before the age of 15 years, with the highest frequency between the ages of 1 and 5 years. The acute phase of the disease starts when *Trypanosoma cruzi* enters the body. A local reaction at the portal of entry is followed by general malaise. All clinical manifestations decline after 4–8 weeks, or less if specific parasiticidal treatment (*2*) is provided.

Most cases of Chagas disease are caused by infected triatomine bugs when they puncture the skin to feed on blood and simultaneously deposit faeces or urine containing trypomastigotes of *T. cruzi*. The itching caused by the bite leads to scratching, allowing the parasites to enter the circulation through the imperceptible wounds thus created. Alternatively, during scratching, parasites can also be transferred to the conjunctiva, where they enter the body even in the absence of any skin lesion.

The skin reaction that occurs at the portal of entry of the parasites is called a chagoma. Triatomine bugs usually bite any part of the body left uncovered during sleep — often the face. Shortly after the triatomine bite, especially if it was close to the eye, a painless reaction of the conjunctiva develops, with unilateral oedema of both eyelids and lymphadenitis of the preauricular ganglia. This is a characteristic sign of acute infection (Romaña's sign) and is an easy way to recognize the disease in endemic areas. Nevertheless, differential diagnosis is necessary to exclude other diseases, such as myiasis, conjunctivitis, ocular traumatism, retroocular thrombosis, or insect bites, which can produce similar signs. A bite in any other part of the skin can give rise to a reaction of the subcutaneous tissue with local oedema and induration, vascular congestion, and cellular infiltration that may quickly be followed by regional lymphadenitis. Fever, polylymphadenopathy, hepatomegaly, and splenomegaly then develop, and may be followed by vomiting, diarrhoea, and anorexia. An electrocardiogram can show signs of heart involvement, such as sinus tachycardia, first-degree atrioventricular (A–V) block, low QRS voltage, or primary T-wave changes. Heart failure can also be observed. Chest X-ray can show cardiomegaly of different degrees. These cardiac abnormalities disappear spontaneously in most cases after 4–8 weeks without any apparent sequelae. In fewer than 3% of acute cases, and mainly in patients under the age of 3 years, this acute myocarditis may have a fatal course.

During this phase, other patients can develop meningoencephalitis with fever, convulsions, and/or loss of consciousness. This severe neurological complication, associated with a mortality of up to 50%, is rare and occurs most often in the second or third year of life.

Acute Chagas disease is recognized only in an estimated 1–2% of all individuals acquiring the infection.

Other ways in which Chagas disease can be acquired and cause an initial acute phase include congenital infection, infection acquired through blood transfusion or organ transplant from an infected donor, oral transmission, and laboratory accident. The most common are infection acquired by blood transfusion and transplacental infection (the so-called congenital form).

Transfusion of blood from an infected donor can produce acute Chagas disease, with clinical manifestations appearing between a few days and several weeks after the transfusion. In these cases, there is no skin reaction at the portal of entry, and most cases are probably asymptomatic. The most frequent clinical sign is fever, but splenomegaly and polylymphadenopathy can also be observed. In addition, generalized oedema and hepatomegaly have been described. The electrocardiogram and the chest X-ray can show the same types of abnormalities as those seen in any other form of acute Chagas disease. Diagnosis is confirmed by direct parasitological tests. However, many cases may go unrecognized since the symptoms produced by this form usually overlap with these of the clinical condition that necessitated the blood transfusion. Moveover, where the latency period is long, the symptoms (most commonly fever) are unlikely to be associated with a blood transfusion performed several weeks earlier, so that the acute phase of the disease is overlooked. While many patients are believed to have received infected blood, only a small number of cases of bloodborne acute Chagas disease have actually been reported. The risk of acquiring the disease in this way is directly related to the number of transfusions received. It is estimated that the risk of transmission as a result of a transfusion from an infected donor may be as high as 25%.

Organ transplant from an infected donor to a non-infected recipient is also a means of transmission of acute Chagas disease, the risk being increased by the immunosuppression required by the procedure. However, this form is epidemiologically irrelevant in endemic areas since the situation is generally recognized in advance and the disease can be prevented by specific treatment.

Oral transmission is a common route of *T. cruzi* circulation in the sylvatic cycle, where several mammals, such as marsupials and primates, eat triatomines and smaller reservoir hosts. In the domestic environment, dogs and cats eat both infected rodents and bugs.

Acute Chagas disease acquired through a laboratory accident is uncommon but potentially dangerous if it goes unnoticed. Clinical manifestations can vary from mild to severe, and the outcome is related to the immunological condition of the patient, the biological characteristics of the *T. cruzi* strain, and the magnitude of the inoculum. If the infected individual becomes aware of the accident in good time, appropriate treatment can avert the infection (see Annex 1).

2.1.2 *Chronic phase*

The chronic phase of Chagas disease starts when parasitaemia falls to undetectable levels and both general symptoms and any clinical manifestations of acute myocarditis or meningoencephalitis disappear. These parasitological and clinical changes usually take place some 4–8 weeks after infection.

In untreated individuals, it is thought that the level of parasitaemia decreases as a consequence of equilibrium being reached between the parasite and the immunological response of the infected individual. This equilibrium can last for the rest of a patient's life, and conventional IgG antibodies against *T. cruzi* can be detected. Parasitological tests, such as xenodiagnosis or haemoculture, can demonstrate circulating parasites in at least half of all infected individuals several years after the original infection took place. Routine clinical procedures reveal no objective evidence of organ damage in such patients; both electrocardiograms and chest X-rays are normal, as is radiology of the oesophagus and colon.

Current knowledge of all the changes produced by the infection during this evolution of the disease is incomplete, and this initial period of the chronic phase is therefore called the indeterminate or latent form of Chagas disease (see below).

Indeterminate form

The acute phase is followed by the indeterminate form of chronic Chagas disease. About 50–70% of infected individuals will remain in this condition for the rest of their lives. Those with the indeterminate form thus account for the vast majority of individuals with the chronic infection. In endemic areas where vectorial transmission still occurs, they act as a natural reservoir of *T. cruzi* infection and contribute to maintaining the life cycle of the parasite.

Most patients with the indeterminate form of the disease are aged 20–50 years, i.e. they are economically productive. They can be identified by epidemiological surveys or by medical or serological examinations such as those performed on blood donors in endemic areas. Their mortality is the same as that of the general population. However, sensitive and specific clinical methods of study often disclose subtle changes in different organs or systems in some patients.

Several studies of autonomic function have demonstrated changes in both the sympathetic and parasympathetic nervous system. Changes have been found in saliva and sweat production, gall-bladder contractility, skin conductance threshold, heart rate, blood pressure control, and oesophageal and gastric pressure. Levels of neurotransmitters such as catecholamines and acetylcholine or related enzymes, as well as of purinergic substances, were found to be changed in patients with the indeterminate form of the disease compared with normal individuals.

Studies of the central nervous system have revealed changes in the somatosensory and auditory evoked potentials of the brain that have been linked to modifications in central myelin. The peripheral nervous system is also affected in chronic chagasic patients. Electromyographic studies have found changes that suggest that Chagas disease causes lesions in the motorneurons of the ventral horn of the spinal cord as well as in the sensory neurons of the dorsal root ganglion. Axonal loss and demyelination of the peripheral nerves have also been described.

Some patients with the chronic indeterminate form and with a normal electrocardiogram, which records only about 1 minute of electrical activity of the myocardium, may show alterations if they undergo ambulatory electrocardiographic monitoring (Holter monitoring) for 24 hours (1440 minutes) while they carry out their normal daily activities (see also p. 8). In this way, changes in heart frequency control and rhythm, and cardiac conduction abnormalities can be detected by comparison with normal controls.

Exercise stress tests, echocardiograms, radionuclide studies, angiography, and His bundle electrograms can also show cardiac abnormalities such as arrhythmias, abnormal wall contractions, coronary arteries with lumen enlargement, and diminished flow velocity or conduction defects not visible on surface electrocardiograms. These alterations can be observed in some asymptomatic individuals with the chronic indeterminate form of Chagas disease whose electrocardiograms and chest X-ray examinations show no abnormalities.

In up to 11% of asymptomatic patients in whom the oesophagus is of normal shape in the X-ray examination, pharmacological or manometric recording of the progression of a barium swallow can expose subtle abnormalities of oesophageal dynamics. No similar surveys of colon physiology with normal barium contrast examinations have been performed in asymptomatic populations due to technical difficulties in carrying them out under field conditions (3).

Not all patients with the chronic indeterminate form of Chagas disease show the same clinical picture. In most, no abnormality can be demonstrated, while in others some functional or organic changes can be detected. Hence, the chronic indeterminate form provides a good opportunity to categorize patients in epidemiological surveys based on the results of serology, electrocardiography, and radiological studies of the heart, oesophagus, and colon. Unfortunately, most epidemiological surveys do not include the use of contrast media in the examination of the oesophagus and colon because of the difficulty of carrying out such tests in the field.

Cardiac form

Chagasic cardiomyopathy is the most important clinical consequence of *T. cruzi* infection. Epidemiological studies show that, among individuals with positive specific serology, about 10–30% have some characteristic changes in their electrocardiogram that indicate cardiac damage caused by the parasite. These changes occur 10–20 years after the acute phase of the disease and include a broad range of types of damage. The clinical manifestations vary from mild symptoms to heart failure and, frequently, sudden death. Inflammation with accompanying fibrosis scattered throughout the myocardium results in severe heart lesions — the cardiac form of chronic Chagas disease. The factors that induce the transition from the indeterminate to the cardiac form of the disease are unknown.

The main clinical manifestations of chronic chagasic cardiomyopathy are heart failure, cardiac arrhythmias, and thromboembolism. Heart failure gives rise to dyspnoea and oedema. As the myocardial lesion involves both right and left ventricles, advanced cases present predominant right ventricle insufficiency, producing oedema and congestive hepatomegaly. Heart enlargement leads to mitral and tricuspid insufficiency. In these dilated hearts, intracavitary right and left ventricular thrombi are often seen and are the principal source of pulmonary embolisms and embolisms in other organs, mainly brain, spleen, and kidney. Cerebral embolism resulting from this dilated cardiomyopathy has been considered to be one of the leading causes of brain ischaemia in endemic zones.

The electrocardiogram almost always shows, either alone or in combination, right bundle branch block, left anterior hemiblock, prolonged A–V conduction time, primary T-wave changes, and abnormal Q waves as the characteristic alterations. Left posterior hemiblock is less frequently seen. As a distinctive feature in the electrocardiographic picture of a cardiomyopathy, left bundle branch block has a remarkably low prevalence.

Arrhythmias are the consequence of both focal and diffusely scattered lesions of the myocardium. Ventricular extrasystoles are the most common arrhythmias and are often almost continuous and multiform; they are isolated, in couplets, or in episodes of ventricular tachycardia of variable duration. Physical effort increases their frequency. Sustained ventricular tachycardia is common even in patients with little or no heart enlargement. Such tachycardia often produces haemodynamic decompensation. Ventricular tachycardias are usually polymorphic, and are sometimes also present as *torsade de pointes*. Either of these two types of tachycardia can degenerate into ventricular fibrillation, which is considered to be the main cause of sudden death.

Arrhythmias can also be bradycardic. Sinus bradycardia is common among chagasic patients, and different degrees of sinoatrial block are also regularly seen. Atrial fibrillation, usually with low ventricular response, is a frequent complication of advanced cases. Atrioventricular block of first, second, or third degree as a consequence of A–V nodal lesions or, most commonly, as a result of the interruption of the intraventricular conduction system leads to low or very low ventricular rhythms requiring permanent pacing. Occasionally, His bundle electrograms are necessary to reveal suspected intraventricular conduction defects that are not visible on the surface electrocardiogram.

Chest X-rays are usually required in the management of these patients since they permit more precise clinical categorization through the evaluation of cardiac size and pulmonary circulation. Physical fitness is studied by means of exercise testing: this standardized test can also show whether a chagasic patient with few, if any, ventricular extrasystoles at rest is at risk of arrhythmia.

As previously mentioned (see p. 6), ambulatory electrocardiographic monitoring — Holter monitoring — can be used to detect cardiac arrhythmias and to study their behaviour, including their frequency and polymorphism. Arrhythmias frequently persist throughout the day, even during the hours of sleep. Several reports have been published of patients dying while wearing a Holter recording device: later analysis of the electrocardiogram showed that ventricular fibrillation was the final event. Echocardiography, radionuclide studies, and angiography can reveal abnormalities in the size of the cavities and in their wall contraction, and can clearly show the apical aneurysm that is characteristic of chagasic cardiomyopathy. Angiography can show dilated coronary arteries in which flow velocity is reduced. In addition, echocardiography — which is routinely used in the evaluation of chagasic patients — often reveals intracavitary thrombi. Cases with severe heart enlargement generally have a very poor prognosis (*4*).

Changes in the peripheral nervous system
In about 10% of patients with chronic Chagas disease, neurological examination shows at least one clinical manifestation of peripheral nervous system damage. Most such patients present a combination of sensory impairment and diminished tendon jerks, mainly affecting the lower limbs.

Sensory abnormalities, such as paraesthesia, and touch and pain hypoaesthesia, are common findings. Sensory impairment in the form of paraesthesia of the lower limbs and/or diminished sensitivity to pinpricks and touch, is one of the commonest manifestations. Impairment of the sense of vibration and of position can also be found. Tendon jerks are diminished in symptomatic patients, either alone or combined with sensory impairment, the most commonly affected being the patellar and Achilles tendon reflexes. Conventional electromyography shows a severely reduced interference pattern. In comparison with uninfected individuals, patients show loss of a number of functional motor units in the tenar and hypotenar groups, the soleus, and the extensor digitorum brevis. No direct relationship is found between cardiac involvement and loss of motor units. Conduction velocity in peripheral motor nerves is slower than the lowest velocity seen in controls. The most important feature of this neuropathy is sensory disturbance. Muscle weakness is not usually observed. Hence, these alterations are not particularly troublesome and do not prevent patients from carrying out their usual activities (5).

Digestive form
The destruction of the autonomic enteric innervation caused by *T. cruzi* infection leads to dysfunction of the digestive system. Both anatomical and functional alterations can be observed at different levels. Abnormalities are most frequently found in the oesophagus and in the colon, apparently because both handle harder material, such as the alimentary bolus and stools.

The digestive form of chronic Chagas disease has been described in all populations south of the Equator. However, striking differences in its prevalence have repeatedly been observed in different countries. In hospital-based observations, mega-oesophagus is more frequently seen than megacolon, probably because dysphagia is a symptom that prompts patients to seek medical care with greater urgency than constipation. Megagastria, megaduodenum, and cholecystomegaly have also been described, always associated with mega-oesophagus and/or megacolon (6).

Mega-oesophagus. As with chronic chagasic cardiomyopathy, estimates of the prevalence of chagasic oesophageal lesions in a population will depend on the screening method used. Manometric or pharmacological investigation may reveal abnormalities in the motility of the oesophagus in an otherwise asymptomatic chagasic individual. However, the radiological method, which is well accepted by patients, is sufficiently sensitive to identify the majority of symptomatic — and even some asymptomatic — cases and is thus adequate for epidemiological surveys. It allows an evaluation of oesophageal transit, of the diameter of the oesophagus, and of the degree of retention of ingested food, as well as of the resting pressure of the lower oesophageal sphincter. Radiological surveys in rural communities have shown that the anectasic form is more prevalent. However, when chagasic individuals are studied in the hospital environment, ectasic forms predominate.

The intrinsic denervation of the oesophagus caused by *T. cruzi* infection results in a loss of oesophageal peristalsis and achalasia of the lower oesophageal sphincter.

From the clinical viewpoint, the extent to which the oesophagus is involved may vary, ranging from slight motor disturbances to the pronounced dilation that characterizes the more advanced forms of mega-oesophagus. A high degree of intrinsic denervation is required for the development of complete aperistalsis and total achalasia of the lower oesophageal sphincter. The symptoms and evolution will therefore depend on the intensity of the anatomical lesions and functional disorders of the oesophagus.

The initial main symptom, almost always present, is dysphagia. With the progression of the disease, this is followed by thoracic pain, active and passive regurgitation, heartburn, hiccups, cough, ptyalism, enlargement of the salivary glands — mainly the parotids — and emaciation. Obstipation is also a common complaint not necessarily related to concomitant megacolon.

An X-ray examination using two films is recommended for detection of cases: the first is taken immediately after the swallowing of 150 ml of a barium contrast medium and the second 1 minute later (even when this second film alone may be enough for practical diagnostic purposes). The following features, observed on the second film, are sufficient for an appropriate diagnosis:

(a) normal diameter of the oesophagus;
(b) incomplete emptying of the oesophagus, with the remaining barium contrast medium forming a cylindrical shape with a horizontal upper level;

(c) the presence of air above the contrast medium along the entire length of the oesophagus.

Even if this technique does not reveal all cases of chagasic oesophagopathy, it will identify cases without dilation. In addition, if features (b) and (c) are carefully evaluated, it will be unlikely that an individual with oesophageal changes will be considered as normal. However, in the differential diagnosis, some conditions that may cause partial retention of the barium meal in the oesophagus should be considered, e.g. presby-oesophagus, systemic sclerosis, tumour of the gastric fundus, stenosis of the cardia, hiatus hernia, reflux oesophagitis, extrinsic compression, and the use of anticholinergic drugs.

Chagasic mega-oesophagus may be divided into four radiological groups, as follows. Group I comprises the anectasic form, while groups II and III are the intermediate forms, with more uncoordinated tertiary contractions and a minor dilation in group II as compared with group III. Group IV includes the most advanced form, the dolichomega-oesophagus.

It has been observed that the prevalence and severity of mega-oesophagus decrease in those regions where transmission control has been successful. Available data indicate a more serious evolution of the disease in males. The conventional electrocardiogram shows that more than 30% of patients with mega-oesophagus have alterations commensurate with chronic chagasic cardiomyopathy. The most frequent electrocardiographic alterations are complete right bundle branch block, with or without left anterior hemiblock, and ventricular extrasystoles (3).

Megacolon. The prevalence of colopathy in endemic areas is unknown because of the practical difficulty of studying it in the field. As an isolated manifestation of Chagas disease, megacolon is infrequent; it is usually associated with mega-oesophagus and/or cardiomyopathy. Dilation occurs mainly in the sigmoid colon and extends to the rectum in about 80% of cases. In a few instances the entire colon may be dilated. Barium enema is the best method of detecting megacolon.

The main signs and symptoms that suggest a diagnosis of megacolon are associated with the retention of faeces and gas. Constipation is the most frequent symptom in patients who seek medical care. However, among non-selected chagasic patients, nearly 25% of those in whom barium enema indicates a colon dilation have normal bowel movements at intervals of less than two days. Furthermore, constipation is a very common condition that may not be related to megacolon. Other frequent symptoms are meteorism, uncomfortable abdominal distension, and sometimes abdominal cramps. In addition, patients complain of difficulty in expelling stools, even when they are of normal consistency. Abdominal examination may reveal the presence of fecaloma, which is easily recognized by its peculiar consistency.

As in mega-oesophagus, manometric studies of the colon have shown motor disorders due to intrinsic denervation. One of the most characteristic motor disturbances in megacolon consists of rectum–sigmoid motor incoordination. Basal motility may be increased or decreased, and there is hypersensitivity to cholinergic stimulation by methacholine or neostigmine.

Another important feature of megacolon physiopathology is achalasia of the internal anal sphincter, which does not relax with distension of the rectum as in normal individuals. Besides the loss of this reflex, there is also hyposensitivity of the rectum wall, a stronger than normal stimulus being necessary to induce the need to defecate.

Many cases of megacolon also present an elongation of the sigmoid colon (dolichomegacolon). Cancer associated with megacolon is rare and, when present, is located in the non-dilated portion of the colon.

Stomach. Intrinsic denervation of the stomach is indicated by alterations in gastric motility and secretion. The stomach, like the oesophagus and the colon, becomes hyperreactive to cholinergic stimuli and its capacity for emptying is altered, being increased for liquids and decreased for solid meals. A large stomach dilation is rare, possibly because of the retention of food by the dilated oesophagus. In cases of advanced mega-oesophagus, a small stomach is a common finding.

Mucosal alterations characteristic of chronic gastritis are frequent. However, apart from denervation, several other factors have been incriminated as causes of chronic gastritis, such as the irritation caused by food that remains in the oesophagus for a long time, duodenogastric biliary reflux, low resistance of the mucosa, and the presence of *Helicobacter pylori*.

Duodenum. Parasympathetic denervation in the duodenum is well documented in both experimentally infected animals and human cases. Dyskinetic alterations may be observed on radiological examination of patients with mega-oesophagus, and pharmacological tests of denervation by cholinergic stimulation may be positive by manometric study in chagasic patients with an otherwise normal duodenum. The duodenum is the third most frequently dilated segment in human Chagas disease, after the oesophagus and the colon. Dilation may be restricted to the duodenal bulb or the duodenal arch, or may be present in the whole organ. Megaduodenum is rarely found as an isolated manifestation, but is nearly always associated with mega-oesophagus and/or megacolon.

Jejunum and ileum.   Radiological studies of the small intestine in patients with mega-oesophagus have demonstrated changes in transit velocity, which may be slower or faster, as well as other alterations of the mucosal surface and of motor activity. The absorption of monosaccharides is accelerated in cases of enteropathy, a finding revealed by an abnormal glucose tolerance test with abnormal increase in glycaemia in the initial phase of the test. The jejunal bacterial flora, both aerobic and anaerobic, is increased in patients with mega-oesophagus, independently of the basal levels of stomach acid secretion. Dilation of the jejunum and ileum, with the appearance of megajejunum and megaileum, is rare.

Extrahepatic biliary tract.   The gall-bladder, like the entire digestive tract, also presents intrinsic denervation in Chagas disease. Functional studies of the gall-bladder by various methods in patients with the digestive form of the disease have shown anomalous responses. Radiological examination has demonstrated hypersensitivity to stimulation by cholecystokinin octapeptide as well as to the endogenous cholecystokinin released by a lipid emulsion introduced into the duodenum. With ultrasound imaging, an accelerated emptying of the gall-bladder under cholinergic stimulation with methacholine and a slow and incomplete emptying after a liquid meal have been observed. Hypertony of Oddi's sphincter and an increase in phasic activity are seen in patients with mega-oesophagus. Cholecystomegaly has been described in up to 4% of patients with megacolon and/or mega-oesophagus. It is not yet clear whether cholecystopathy favours lithogenesis: published data are contradictory. However, it has been reported that cholelithiasis is more prevalent in chronic patients with the cardiac form of the disease than in the general population. Moreover, the incidence of cholelithiasis appears to be higher in patients with mega-oesophagus than in those with the cardiac or indeterminate form of Chagas disease.

Congenital form
Congenital Chagas disease is produced by the transmission of *T. cruzi* from the infected mother to the child. The risk factors that may

determine whether a pregnant woman will give birth to an infected child have not been defined. Infection of the fetus may occur at any time during pregnancy and in different pregnancies of the same woman. In the case of twins, *T. cruzi* may infect just one fetus or both. Abortion is uncommon. Most infected pregnant women will not transmit the infection to their offspring: the incidence of congenital transmission in general varies from 1 to 10% in different geographical zones, even within the same country.

Most infected infants are asymptomatic and have normal weight and vital signs, but some — mainly those born prematurely — may show a broad spectrum of clinical manifestations, such as low body weight for gestational age, jaundice, anaemia, hepatomegaly, splenomegaly, symptoms of meningoencephalitis and/or myocarditis, as well as ocular lesions. Prognosis is poor in such cases. In areas where vector control has been successful, there is a marked tendency for the incidence of congenital Chagas disease to decline because of the decreasing numbers, or even a total absence, of infected fertile young women (7).

Immunosuppressed host
The growing use of immunosuppressive drugs to prevent the rejection of transplanted solid organs and bone marrow, as well as the increase in immunosuppression as a result of lymphoproliferative diseases and AIDS, has increased the risk of reactivation of chronic Chagas disease or *T. cruzi* transmission through infected grafts or bone marrow donations (see also section 6.1.4).

The most important clinical symptoms and signs reported in association with Chagas disease and the immunosuppression associated with transplantation or AIDS are panniculitis, central nervous system lesions, meningoencephalitis, and myocarditis.

Infected as well as non-infected individuals who have received solid organs or bone marrow from infected donors must be given specific treatment and appropriate follow-up in order to prevent transmission. All recipients, whether serologically reactive or non-reactive, of a graft or bone marrow from donors infected with *T. cruzi* must be checked for parasitaemia every week for 2 months after transplantation, every 15 days during the third month, and every month during the entire period of pharmacological immunosuppression. Early diagnosis of subclinical disease and the timely use of trypanosomicidal therapy are essential in the follow-up of patients who have undergone any type of transplant (8).

Kidney transplantation. Early reports of Chagas disease associated with transplantation in the Americas concerned patients who had received kidney transplants, and described a fatal evolution usually resulting from infection acquired through blood transfusion during the transplant. In the 1980s and early 1990s, it was reported that chronic chagasic patients who underwent immunosuppression in connection with kidney transplantation, or lymphoproliferative or autoimmune disease did not show reactivation of the disease. At that time, it seemed that immunosuppression was not able to upset the delicate balance between the parasite and the immune response in the infected host. However, recent reports indicate that reactivation, as shown by detectable parasitaemia, as well as *T. cruzi* transmission through the graft, is possible. The incidence of both phenomena varies between countries. The critical time for the appearance of clinical and laboratory manifestations of reactivation or infection was 2–5 months after transplantation, with exceptional cases appearing as late as 2 or more years afterwards. However, other studies have found that reactivation occurs between 7 days and 14 months after transplantation. Careful monitoring allows early diagnosis and antiparasitic treatment with the possibility of full recovery.

Heart transplantation. The survival time and quality of life of patients with advanced chronic Chagas disease who receive a heart transplant do not seem to differ from those of patients suffering from other cardiomyopathies, so that heart transplantation is a therapeutic option for patients with advanced chagasic cardiomyopathy. Reactivation of the disease in an infected recipient is possible as a consequence of the necessary immunosuppression, but lowering the dosage of immunosuppressors reduces the risk. Specific antiparasitic treatment should be considered after heart transplantation. Periodic surveillance for possible parasitaemia is essential; if it occurs, the necessary treatment should be given (*9*).

Bone marrow transplantation. Less than half of the infected patients who receive an allogenic bone marrow transplant show reactivation of the disease. No reactivation has been detected in autologous bone marrow transplantation. Chagasic patients receiving this type of transplantation must be carefully followed up to detect potential reactivation and treated if necessary. Similarly, when bone marrow is obtained from an infected patient, the donor must receive specific antiparasitic treatment before the material is taken for transplantation (*10*).

Liver transplantation. There has been little experience of this type of transplantation associated with Chagas disease, but there seem to be no contraindications for the procedure in recipients with chronic Chagas disease. However, transplantation of a liver from an infected donor to a serologically negative patient would be acceptable only in a clinical emergency.

Pancreas, lung, corneal, and vascular grafts, and other types of transplant. There is no information on these types of transplants associated with Chagas disease, but it is generally agreed that patients infected with *T. cruzi* can receive them. On the other hand, infected donors are accepted even for negative receptors only in extreme cases.

Oncohaematological and autoimmune disorders. There is some evidence that Chagas disease can be reactivated in patients with leukaemia and lymphoma, but reactivation has not been documented in patients with autoimmune disorders.

AIDS. Reactivation of Chagas disease in patients with AIDS has been well documented, mainly when CD4 lymphocytes are below $200/mm^3$. The two most frequent localizations were the central nervous system and the heart, and specific antiparasitic treatment is then required. Although the prevention of reactivation by trypanocidal therapy has been suggested, the general adoption of treatment by means of a cocktail of antiretroviral drugs has made the reactivation of Chagas disease in AIDS patients unlikely, since the treatment restores the level of CD4 lymphocytes to the normal value.

Serological criteria for the acceptance or rejection of transplants. Based on the available data, the serological criteria for the acceptance or rejection of transplants are shown in Table 1. All recipients with positive serology should be accepted for organ or bone marrow transplantation except in the case of heart transplants from positive donors. The use of both dead and living donors with positive serology for negative recipients is also accepted for kidney transplants in endemic areas. Other solid organ transplants should be accepted only in extreme cases. In the case of bone marrow transplants, infected donors may be accepted in spite of the lack of data on the outcome, given the difficulty of finding histocompatible donors. However, antiparasitic treatment must be administered when positive donors are used in order to reduce the potential parasite inoculation through an infected organ or bone marrow. Informed consent is al-

Table 1
Serological criteria for the acceptance or rejection of transplants

Organ	Donor	Recipient	Recommendation
Kidney from cadaver	Positive	Positive	Acceptance
	Positive	Negative	Acceptance
Kidney from living donor	Positive	Positive	Acceptance
	Positive	Negative	Acceptance
Heart	Negative	Positive	Acceptance
	Positive	Positive	Rejection
	Positive	Negative	Rejection
Liver (emergency)	Positive	Positive	Acceptance
	Positive	Negative	Acceptance
Liver (urgency)	Positive	Positive	Acceptance
	Positive	Negative	Rejection
Liver (elective)	Positive	Positive	Acceptance
	Positive	Negative	Rejection
Bone marrow	Positive	Positive	Acceptance
	Positive	Negative	Acceptance

ways an essential requirement before the procedure is carried out, and strict post-transplantation monitoring is mandatory.

It is worth mentioning that, in some Chagas disease recipients of kidney or bone marrow transplants, previously positive serological reactivity was turned to negative during immunosuppression. However, in these cases parasitaemia can occur with or without discernible clinical signs of Chagas disease. This suggests that exhaustive screening for the parasite might be more appropriate than serology in the diagnosis of the reactivation of chronic Chagas disease. While the presence of Chagas disease should not be regarded as a contraindication in solid organ and bone marrow transplantation, persons with positive serology must be carefully studied and treated with benznidazole before they can be considered as candidates for donation. This requirement is based on the fact that subclinical parasitaemia in chronic chagasic patients is frequently missed by the parasitological detection methods currently in use.

2.2 Pathology

2.2.1 *Acute phase*

Lesions at the portal of entry are similar whether they occur in the conjunctiva or in the subcutaneous tissue. Early reactions are mainly nonspecific and include vascular congestion, oedema, and peripheral leukocyte infiltrations; later, lymphocytes and monocytes predominate, and later still, an invasion of the tissues by fibroblasts, giant cells, and lymphocytes may be observed. When a biopsy of satellite nodes has been made, the lesions have been compatible with an acute nonspecific adenitis with proliferation of hystiocytes in the sinusoids; multinucleated giant cells, with or without parasites, may sometimes be seen.

The pathology of the heart may vary from no alterations in the heart muscle fibres to muscle cells parasitized with amastigotes, with or without a peripheral inflammatory reaction. Findings have included muscle fibres full of parasites with signs of myocitolysis, penetration of macrophages into the fibres, free parasites or macrophages with phagocytized parasites, and infiltration of lymphocytes, monocytes, and/or polymorphonuclear cells and sometimes eosinophils.

The histopathological lesions of the nervous system are those of acute meningoencephalitis. The meninges show vascular congestion, haemorrhagic microfoci, and inflammatory infiltration with polymorphonuclear cells, lymphocytes, plasmocytes, and macrophages, with or without amastigotes. Parasites may be found free in the perivascular spaces or nestled within the glia or neuronal cells. Similar tissue manifestations may also be found in the cerebellum and in the medulla.

2.2.2 *Chronic phase: heart pathology*

Indeterminate form
Pathological studies of the chronic indeterminate form are scarce and inconclusive. In most of the few published autopsy studies of chagasic patients dying from causes — mainly violent — other than Chagas disease no clinical information was available from which a patient's condition could be accurately identified as the chronic indeterminate form. As patients with this form of the disease are asymptomatic, such methodological flaws are unavoidable.

Another way to study the pathological changes in patients with the chronic indeterminate form of the disease is through endomyocardial biopsy. This in vivo procedure has the advantage of providing precise diagnosis. However, the material obtained is from limited zones of the endocardium and is not representative of the whole cardiac mass.

In the indeterminate form, mild multifocal myocarditis can be observed. It appears as scattered small foci of interstitial inflammatory cell infiltration by lymphocytes, macrophages, and plasma cells in the myocardium, lacking the intimate association with degenerating myocytes observed during the acute phase of the disease, and sometimes disclosing a granulomatous structure. Changes can also involve the conducting tissue of the heart (*11*).

Material obtained through endomyocardial biopsies has allowed the application of more refined techniques such as electron microscopy, histochemistry, and immunohistochemistry. Light and electron microscopic studies of such biopsies have revealed myocyte hypertrophy, degenerative changes, inflammation, and fibrosis in some patients with the chronic indeterminate form of Chagas disease. Myocytes are enlarged, with prominent and hyperchromatic nuclei. Atrophic and degenerating myocytes show lipofuscin pigmentation, evidence of cell membrane alterations, and vacuolization of the cytoplasm. Ultrastructural changes include several degrees of mitochondrial oedema and atrophy, and incipient dilatation of T tubules with intratubular deposits of microfilaments of a glycoprotein-like substance. The inflammatory cells infiltrating cardiac tissues consist of lymphocytes, plasma cells, macrophages, and a few mast cells. Small scars and patches of interstitial fibrous tissue surrounding atrophic myocardial fibres are occasionally present.

Intact tissue parasites are rarely found, but the persistence of *T. cruzi* DNA can be demonstrated in the myocardium of these patients by the polymerase chain reaction (PCR), even in the absence of local inflammation. Longitudinal studies have demonstrated that mild focal myocardial lesions are not cumulative and the uninvolved myocardium usually appears normal.

Cardiac form
The inflammatory cell reaction observed in the chronic phase of Chagas disease has recently been characterized as consisting mainly of cytotoxic CD8+ T lymphocytes (*12*). It is generally agreed that these lymphocytes are the main T-cell type responsible for immune activation in chronic chagasic cardiomyopathy. These cells are activated, through class I major histocompatibility complex (MHC) molecules, by macrophages containing remnants of *T. cruzi*. The absence of a CD4+ T-cell response in the presence of *T. cruzi* antigens suggests that the presentation of these antigens through class II MHC molecules is inhibited (*13, 14*). However, experimental evidence suggests that depletion of CD4+ lymphocytes in the chronic phase of Chagas disease is related to selective apoptosis of these cells (*15*).

In advanced cases of cardiomegaly, signs of chronic passive congestion and thromboembolic phenomena are the main gross pathological findings. Cardiomegaly is due to a combination of hypertrophy, dilatation, and alteration of the heart muscle architecture; the weight of the heart is usually increased. Apical cardiac aneurysm is a frequent finding and is pathognomonic of chronic chagasic cardiomyopathy. Focal areas of myocardial atrophy occur at random in the myocardium.

Endocardial mural thrombi occur frequently in necropsies, accompanied by infarctus in several organs such as the lungs, kidneys, spleen, and brain. Chagasic heart disease is thus an embolizing condition. Chronic diffuse myocarditis with marked interstitial fibrosis is seen microscopically.

Myocyte changes include hypertrophy, necrosis, and degenerative abnormalities such as vacuolization, accumulation of lipofuscin granules, hyaline degeneration, intracellular oedema, and disruption and loss of myofibrils. Hypertrophic myocytes display enlarged and hyperchromatic nuclei but may exhibit attenuation (stretching) in dilated hearts. Full necrosis is best appreciated in foci where inflammatory cells appear to be inside myocardial fibres (abscessed myocytes). Atrophic myocytes are commonly present in the dense patches of fibrous tissue. A combination of hypertrophic and atrophic myocardial fibres against a background of a chronic active and fibrosing myocarditis is highly suggestive of *T. cruzi* etiology.

Ultrastructural observations show several degrees of regressive changes in myocardiocytes, such as mitochondrial swelling with cristae disruption, accumulation of glycogen particles, or thickening of the basement membrane as well as in myocardial capillaries. These changes may interfere with the metabolism and diffusion of nutrients to contractile fibres.

Amastigote forms of *T. cruzi* are rarely found in histological sections when standard techniques are used. When amastigote forms are identified in the cytoplasm of myocardial cells, no reaction is observed in the tissues surrounding intact parasitized myocytes. Disrupted parasitized myocytes are characteristically infiltrated by polymorphonuclear cells, eosinophils, macrophages, and lymphocytes (abscessed myofibres), which extend beyond the limits of the affected foci.

Immunochemistry greatly improves the level of detection of intact intracellular amastigotes. With this technique, intramyocardial parasites were demonstrated in biopsies of chronic chagasic patients; these were also observed when PCR and in-situ hybridization were used to demonstrate the presence of *T. cruzi* in the tissues (*16–18*). Degenerative and fibrotic changes occur in the conducting tissue. Lesions are the same as those found in the contractile myocardium.

2.2.3 *Chronic phase: digestive form*

The study of different segments of the digestive tract shows focal myositis and unevenly distributed lesions of the intramural plexuses, mainly the myenteric plexus. Jejunal neuronal lesions are less pronounced than those found in the oesophagus and colon. The remaining neuronal cells have alterations suggestive of neurotransmitter hypersecretion as a compensation mechanism for denervation. The common anatomical abnormality underlying this form of the disease is the destruction of parasympathetic ganglion cells associated with the muscular layers of the dilated organs. Nerve destruction usually develops insidiously, but the exact mechanism of neuronolysis is unknown. Histopathological studies of patients with chronic disease have demonstrated inflammation and neuronal depletion in the myenteric plexuses of the oesophagus associated with myositis and fibrosis in the muscularis propria. Parasites are detectable only rarely in these tissues, but the demonstration of distinct *T. cruzi* kinetoplast DNA suggests the intervention of the parasite in the development of chronic lesions in this clinical form of the disease (*19*).

Mega-oesophagus and megacolon associated with *T. cruzi* infection have no morphological features that could be used to differentiate them from sporadically observed idiopathic cases. However, unlike Hirschsprung's disease, the disappearance of neurons from Auerbach's plexus is not limited to the distal non-dilated portion of the colon in the chagasic megacolon. In "mega" conditions associated with *T. cruzi* infection, focal inflammatory lesions may be present in the muscular coat or along the myoenteric plexus. When present, they are represented by lymphocytes, macrophages, and plasma cells distributed in isolated clusters. There is no cell destruction and/or proliferation of vascular and connective cells, so that the infiltration is minimal. Within and around Auerbach's plexus, fibrosis, atrophy of neuronal structures, and total or partial absence of neurons may be observed. When destruction of neurons is only partial, some sort of serial or stepped sectioning and the application of quantitative or morphometric analysis are absolutely necessary to detect neuronal loss. Intracellular amastigotes are rarely found in the muscular fibres of the oesophagus or the colon. In early stages of the disease, hypertrophy of the muscular coat and the muscularis mucosae is prominent, but is replaced by atrophy and dilatation as the disease progresses.

2.2.4 *Chagas disease and AIDS*

A predominant and sometimes exclusive involvement of the central nervous system has been observed in chagasic patients with AIDS. Focal lesions in the brain tend to assume a tumour-like pattern, with accumulation of macrophages loaded with *T. cruzi* amastigotes. Areas of focal necrosis and features of severe meningoencephalitis may also be present. Parasite-induced changes in other organs, including the heart, are mild or nonexistent. The reason for this peculiar tropism of the parasite to the central nervous system in patients with AIDS or certain other immunodeficiencies is not yet understood (*20*).

2.2.5 *Pathogenesis of chronic lesions*

Two main hypotheses have been formulated to explain the pathogenesis of Chagas disease: (1) *T. cruzi* infection induces immune responses which are targeted at self-tissues and are independent of the persistence of the parasite (autoimmunity hypothesis); and (2) the persistence of the parasite at specific sites in tissues of the infected host results in chronic inflammatory reactivity (parasite persistence hypothesis). In both cases, the immune-based pathology results in the cumulative, focal destruction of tissues, and the signs and symptoms of clinical disease.

For a long time, the prevailing hypothesis was that Chagas disease had an autoimmune etiology. This reaction could result either from a loss of tolerance of the immune system to self-antigens induced by chronic *T. cruzi* infection, or tissue lesions could be produced by an immune response elicited by parasite antigens with cross-reactivity against host components (molecular mimicry).

The first reports of the existence of antigens shared by *T. cruzi* and mammalian cells and their role in the pathogenesis of Chagas disease were published in the 1970s and 1980s. Evidence was provided of the existence of antibodies against endothelial cells, vascular endothelium, and heart interstitium (EVI antibodies); laminin; nervous cells; and cardiac sarcoplasmic reticulum (*21*). Human antibodies against parasite ribosomal P proteins were shown to react with self-proteins. Anti-P antibodies have been found in patients with chronic chagasic cardiomyopathy, dilated cardiomyopathy, ventricular arrythmias, and sinus node dysfunction (*22*). In addition, antibodies against an epitope of human cardiac myosin have been reported in patients with chagasic cardiomyopathy (*23*).

Abnormalities of the β-adrenergic and muscarinic cholinergic receptors at post-synaptic levels have been found in patients with chronic Chagas heart disease. These receptor abnormalities may be caused by autoantibodies and induce changes at the level of post-synaptic receptor proteins such as adenylate cyclase, guanylate cyclase, or nitric oxide synthetase (*21*, *24–26*). These changes interfere with the autonomic regulation of the heart and the harmonic muscle contraction of the oesophagus and colon when the disease affects these organs. In addition, in infected organs, the mononuclear cell infiltrate and peripheral lymphocytes release cytokines and biologically active lipid metabolites.

The finding that autoantibodies are present before cardiomyopathy develops may be an indication that they can be an early marker of heart autonomic dysfunction. In fact, circulating β-adrenergic and muscarinic cholinergic antibodies increase with time from infection. Using enzyme-linked immunosorbent assay (ELISA) and a synthetic peptide derived from the second extracellular loop of human β-adrenoceptor and M_2 muscarinic acetylcholine receptor as antigen, a strong association between the presence of circulating antipeptide antibodies in chagasic patients and that of dysautonomic alterations was found. This observation suggests that these autoantibodies may represent a potential marker of autoimmune neurocardiomyopathy. Although supported by experimental data, the autoimmune theory does not explain the multifocal nature of human cardiomyopathy.

The introduction of new techniques such as immunohistochemistry, PCR and in-situ hybridization has provided indisputable evidence of parasite persistence in tissues obtained from patients in the chronic phase of Chagas disease. When an immunoperoxidase technique was used, parasite antigens were detected in the heart of patients with chronic chagasic cardiomyopathy (27). An association between the presence of *T. cruzi* and a moderate or severe inflammatory infiltrate was observed in lesions localized in the basal and posterior walls of the left ventricle.

T. cruzi DNA was consistently detected by PCR in heart specimens from patients with chronic chagasic cardiomyopathy but not in heart tissues from seropositive cadavers without evidence of chagasic cardiopathy (18). It was also found in oesophageal tissue from seropositive patients with mega-oesophagus but not in specimens from patients who died of chronic chagasic cardiomyopathy without mega-oesophagus (19).

Apparently, the different clinical forms of Chagas disease are unrelated to the level of parasitaemia. It is known from experimental studies and from acute human infection that *T. cruzi*, like other parasitic infective agents, induces alterations in the immunological system of the host to circumvent host defence mechanisms. In addition, it has been demonstrated that *T. cruzi* reduces the expression of the lymphocyte surface molecules CD3+, CD4+, and CD8+, which may favour its own survival (28). In myocardial biopsies from chronic chagasic cardiomyopathy, it is possible to observe T cells (96%), most of which are CD8+ T cells, while CD4+ T cells are less frequently seen (27, 29). The number of CD8+ T cells increases in the presence of both scarce and abundant *T. cruzi* antigens, while the number of CD4+ T cells remains unchanged. These findings may suggest that *T. cruzi* antigens play a role in the development of chronic myocarditis, and that a certain degree of immunosuppression permitting parasite survival is also present.

The different clinical and pathological manifestations of human Chagas disease appear to be related to variations in the efficiency of the immune response. In this respect, efficient immune responses control the level of parasitaemia and thus limit tissue damage, while inefficient responses fail to adequately control the parasite burden, thus promoting more persistent inflammatory reactions and more severe disease. It has been suggested that immune responses during the acute phase play a fundamental role in the outcome of chronic manifestations. In addition, differences in parasite strains are another important factor to be considered in the pathogenesis of the disease.

Recent experimental, histological, and clinical observations tend to show that Chagas disease should be regarded mainly as a parasitic infection rather than as an exclusively autoimmune disease. One of the consequences of this pathogenic interpretation is that it may be possible to achieve a favourable outcome in infected patients by the administration of specific parasiticidal treatment.

2.3 Laboratory diagnosis

2.3.1 *Parasitological diagnosis*

During the acute phase of Chagas disease, a large number of parasites are present in peripheral blood and can be detected by direct parasitological tests. For this purpose, the microscopical observation of fresh blood between slide and coverslip can easily disclose the presence of the parasite because of its motility.

Thin and thick blood smears, adequately stained, allow the observation of the morphological characteristics of the parasite, and thus make it possible to differentiate *T. cruzi* from *T. rangeli*. When the level of parasitaemia is low, however, it is necessary to use parasite concentration methods, such as the Strout method and the microhaematocrit.

Xenodiagnosis and haemoculture (possible only in specialized laboratories) are classical indirect parasitological methods whose sensitivity depends on the level of parasitaemia of the individual concerned. Artificial xenodiagnosis has now been developed and may be recommended instead of natural xenodiagnosis. It should be emphasized that, in regions and countries where vectorial transmission has been interrupted, the triatomine species that were the targets of the control programmes should be handled with care to avoid any accidental escape of laboratory insects.

With the advent of molecular techniques, PCR has been used in the parasitological diagnosis of various diseases. This technique relies on the amplification of DNA target sequences, which are both abundant and specific to the parasite concerned. For *T. cruzi*, two target sequences have proved useful in diagnosis: the variable region of the minicircle kinetoplast DNA and a 195-bp reiterated DNA sequence of the parasite (*30*).

Because of the complexity of PCR procedures, this type of diagnosis should be performed only in specialized laboratories. The sensitivity of the technique is higher than that of xenodiagnosis and haemoculture. However, this sensitivity also depends on the level of parasitaemia of the individual. Another important application of PCR is in the detection of parasites in the tissues of chronically infected individuals (*17*, *18*) and in congenital transmission (*31*).

2.3.2 *Immunodiagnosis*

Immunodiagnosis is widely used since nearly all *T. cruzi*-infected individuals in the chronic phase develop antibodies against the complex antigenic mixture of the parasite. In the chronic phase, antibodies are predominantly of the IgG class; in the acute phase, IgM antibodies are found more frequently.

Several diagnostic tests are available, some of which are regarded as conventional; they have been extensively validated, are available on the market, and are used in most laboratories. However, certain tests that are still undergoing testing have better specificity, and some of them may have a number of operational advantages (*32*).

Conventional serology tests

Three conventional tests are widely used: indirect haemagglutination (IHA), indirect immunofluorescence (IIF) and ELISA. It has been suggested that, if positive results are obtained in more than one of the above-mentioned tests, this can be regarded as a definitive diagnosis of *T. cruzi* infection. However, a single positive test, whether IIF or ELISA, should now be sufficient since the sensitivity of these tests is around 99%, provided that the reagents have been subjected to quality controls and stored under the prescribed conditions, and that standard technical procedures have been followed.

In most conventional tests, a complex mixture of parasite antigens (IHA and ELISA) or the entire parasite (IIF) is employed. This increases the likelihood that the infection will be diagnosed, even when the antibody level is low. On the other hand, the chances of false-positive results increase, due to the presence of cross-reactions between *T. cruzi* and *Leishmania* spp. or *T. rangeli*.

An ideal serological test should be easy to perform in a single step, fast, cheap, require no special equipment or refrigeration of reagents, and have a sensitivity and specificity of 100%. Such a test does not exist. However, the conventional tests do have some of these attributes. With the IHA test, results can be obtained in about 2 hours, and no sophisticated equipment or specialized technical skills are needed. The sensitivity attained is in the range of 96–98%, which is lower than that obtained with IIF and ELISA. The test usually fails to detect 1.6–2.5% of infected individuals (false negatives).

The IIF test has a sensitivity of 99% but has several disadvantages: the reading is subjective and must be performed by a skilled technician; a special UV light microscope is needed; and several steps are required. Titration of conjugates is essential as is control of the reagents used. Commercial kits are not readily available, and the specificity is lower than that of the IHA test. False-positive diagnoses cause problems in deciding whether patients and blood donors are infected. The test takes about 2 hours for a few samples. IIF is therefore suitable for small laboratories where a microscope is used for the diagnosis of other infections and where no more than 50–100 samples are tested per day. In blood banks where a larger number of samples are screened, IIF is not recommended.

ELISA has excellent sensitivity and good specificity. As in the case of IIF, it requires a skilled technician and takes several hours to carry out. It has two main advantages compared with IIF: it requires a spectrophotometer, which avoids subjectivity, and it can be automated. ELISA can therefore be used in large centres for the simultaneous screening of many samples. As with other tests, even when different kits are used, borderline results may be obtained. This is a problem in blood banks and also in establishing the etiological diagnosis of a patient.

Considerable expertise has been acquired in recent years with the above-mentioned three tests for the diagnosis of Chagas disease in many countries of Central and South America, and these are the tests that should be used. In 95% of sera, concordant results are obtained with all three tests. When two of the tests disagree, this may indicate technical error or the presence of an unusual serum. Such problems are usually solved by repeating the tests, but if discordant results are still obtained, the serum is problematic and should be given special attention. If this happens in a blood bank, the donor should be excluded. If the problem arises in clinical diagnosis, non-conventional tests (see below) should be used or the serum should be sent to a reference laboratory. In any case, if a serum is repeatedly positive by one test, it should be considered positive.

Antibodies can also be detected by conventional serology in the acute phase of Chagas disease. The IIF test with an anti-IgM conjugate is recommended, although IgG antibodies can also be detected. In congenital transmission, provided that parasites are not found in the blood of the newborn, conventional serology can be performed 6–8 months after delivery, by which time maternal antibodies passively transmitted to the child should have disappeared. The same serological tests can be used for the follow-up of patients undergoing chemotherapy. These recommendations are summarized in Table 2.

Non-conventional serology tests
Some of these tests are already available on the market, but the majority can be obtained only from their producers, mainly universities and research institutes. They are based on ELISA techniques but use reagents such as recombinant proteins, purified antigens, or synthetic peptides. These reagents were developed with the aim of increasing the specificity of the serological diagnosis and avoiding cross-reactivity with other parasitic diseases such as mucocutaneous and visceral leishmaniasis. New matrices have been proposed for use in antigen immobilization, such as strips, coloured beads, and Western blots. The tests most frequently used are those that employ recombinant antigens and have been validated in multicentre trials (*33*).

Recombinant proteins may be used individually or — better — as mixtures of two or more components (*34*). It should be pointed out that, although most of the non-conventional tests show high specificity, their sensitivity may be lower than that of conventional serology. If the results of the two classes of tests are not in agreement, it is recommended that those of the conventional tests should be taken as correct.

A definite advantage of some of the non-conventional tests is their simplicity (one step) and the short time required for execution. The sole disadvantage is that some of the test kits that use strips or beads give only qualitative results.

Table 2
Laboratory diagnosis of Chagas disease

Objectives	Serological and molecular methods				
	Conventional			Non-conventional	
	ELISA	IIF	IHA	Recombinant antigens	PCR
Serological evidence (two tests recommended)	X	X	X	X	
Blood-bank screening (one test recommended)	X				
Transplacental and perinatal transmission (two tests recommended)	X	X		X	X
Epidemiological surveys (one test recommended)	X	X			
Treatment follow-up (two tests recommended)	X	X	X		X

Different procedures can be adopted for the diagnosis of *T. cruzi* infection depending on the situation (see also Table 2), as follows:

- To confirm a clinical suspicion, two conventional tests should be used. If the results are not in agreement, a third test should be performed, either conventional or non-conventional.
- For blood-bank screening, ELISA is recommended.
- With congenital transmission, one conventional test on the mother should be performed, and a positive result confirmed by another conventional test. In children of seropositive mothers, a conventional IgG test should be done 8 months after birth. Parasitological tests are desirable wherever these can be carried out.
- In epidemiological surveys, a single conventional test should be used. Sera, plasma, or blood collected on filter paper can all be used for this purpose.
- In treatment follow-up, two serological tests are recommended. In specialized centres, PCR assays may be performed to verify parasitaemia.

Compliance with good laboratory practice, including the implementation of quality control procedures and periodical evaluation of laboratory performance, together with legislation requiring reagents to be evaluated before they are marketed, is the only way to ensure that the results of serological diagnosis are correct.

2.4 Clinical management and treatment

2.4.1 *Trypanosomicidal treatment*

Nifurtimox (a nitrofuran derivative) and benznidazole (a nitroimi-dazole) have been almost the only drugs used for the treatment of the acute phase of Chagas disease and of congenital infection. Because, until recently, chronic Chagas disease was considered to be an au-toimmune disease, it was generally agreed that patients with overt chronic lesions did not benefit from trypanosomicidal treatment.

This is no longer believed to be true, since it has been shown that benznidazole, when administered to schoolchildren in the chronic phase of the disease, turns to negative up to 60% of previously posi-tive conventional serological tests. Moreover, few children in the benznidazole-treated group developed heart damage when compared with a control group (*35, 36*) (see also p. 34).

Particularly impressive results were obtained in one long-term follow-up study of 131 individuals with chronic cardiomyopathy examined nearly a decade after treatment with benznidazole (*37*). This study found a significant decrease in clinical deterioration in treated as compared with untreated patients. The reduced severity of the dis-ease was also associated with decreased titres of anti-*T. cruzi* anti-bodies, suggesting parasitological cure.

Benznidazole produces side-effects in most adult patients, but these usually disappear when the treatment is discontinued. In only a few cases must treatment be interrupted because of such side-effects. On the other hand, children have a markedly higher tolerance of the treatment.

The general benefits provided by benznidazole in the acute and chronic phases of Chagas disease indicate that treatment with this drug should be recommended for any individual with positive serology (*38*).

The results of several trials carried out in humans to assess the effi-cacy of allopurinol have indicated that this drug lacks any demon-strable parasiticidal activity.

2.4.2 *Drug development*

Although benznidazole is an effective drug for the treatment of Chagas disease, there is a need for new drugs that can be administered for shorter periods and have fewer or no side-effects so as to increase treatment efficacy.

The costs of drug development in the pharmaceutical industry have escalated in recent years. As a consequence, pharmaceutical companies have focused their research and development on areas in which returns will be commensurate with investments. The result has been the complete withdrawal of the major companies from activities directed towards the discovery and development of drugs for tropical diseases (39). On the other hand, the close relationship between *T. cruzi* and other parasites (*T. brucei* group, *Leishmania* spp.) that cause diseases of human and veterinary importance, and their similar susceptibility to a number of drugs already available, may facilitate the development of anti-*T. cruzi* drugs that may also be active against other protozoa. Similarly, the knowledge already gained concerning possible novel targets in trypanosomes that have counterparts in other pathogens or in cancer cells may encourage pharmaceutical companies to develop new drugs for the treatment of Chagas disease. Thus sterol biosynthesis inhibitors, protein prenylation pathway inhibitors (see p. 31), protease inhibitors, and phospholipid analogues are important potential chemotherapeutic agents for this purpose. An additional advantage of some of these compounds, e.g. some sterol biosynthesis inhibitors, for the future of Chagas disease chemotherapy is that they are being developed for a number of different indications (e.g. mycoses).

Sterol metabolism
Azole-containing compounds have provided a major breakthrough in antifungal therapy in both human and veterinary medicine. These drugs interfere with sterol biosynthesis and, together with some other nitrogen heterocycle-containing antifungals, belong to the class of ergosterol biosynthesis inhibitors. Since *T. cruzi* contains ergosterol, it was not unexpected that, when two of these inhibitors, namely miconazole and econazole, were initially tested against this parasite, they showed a potent growth inhibitory action. Later studies showed that ketoconazole and itraconazole were also effective in protecting mice against lethal infections with *T. cruzi* by inhibiting intracellular multiplication of the parasites, and blocking the biosynthesis of sterols. However, although these compounds strongly suppressed *T. cruzi* proliferation in vitro, they failed to achieve parasitological cure in infected experimental animals and in humans.

An important development in this field was the recent demonstration that fourth-generation azole derivatives, such as D0870 and SCH56592 (posaconazole), are capable of achieving parasitological cure in murine models of both acute and chronic Chagas disease (40). The bis-triazole derivative D0870 is a powerful in vitro growth inhibitor of both epimastigotes and intracellular amastigotes, with minimal inhibitory concentrations. In mice, the drug was 30–50 times more powerful than nifurtimox and more than 60% of the animals were parasitologically cured (*41*). Unfortunately, the development of this compound was discontinued in 1997 for toxicological reasons. However, the therapeutic efficacy of posaconazole in animal models has been studied (*41, 42*).

Protein prenylation
The occurrence of protein prenylation in *T. cruzi* and *T. brucei* has been demonstrated. Protein prenylation in mammals and yeast involves the attachment of 15-carbon farnesyl or 20-carbon geranyl-geranyl groups to the C-terminal cysteine residues of a subset of cellular proteins that have roles in cellular signal transduction and intracellular vesicle trafficking. In recent years, hundreds of potent prenylation inhibitors have been synthesized with the primary goal of developing anticancer drugs. Some of these compounds have been shown to inhibit the activity of *T. brucei* recombinant farnesyl transferase and to inhibit the growth of *T. brucei* and *T. cruzi*. Bisphosphonates inhibit the prenylation of small proteins that control cytoskeletal reorganization and apoptosis. Recent studies have shown that bisphosphonates are active in vitro and in vivo against *T. cruzi*.

Proteases
The success of aspartyl protease inhibitors in the chemotherapy of HIV infection has stimulated interest in this type of drug. The use of inhibitors of cystein proteases in animal models of parasitic infections has provided evidence that drugs could be developed to target this class of enzymes.

Phospholipid signalling
The recent success of miltefosine (hexadecylphosphocholine) as a new oral agent for the treatment of visceral leishmaniasis and the demonstration of a suppressive effect of this compound on *T. cruzi* infections have stimulated interest in similar compounds previously shown to have antiviral and anticancer activities.

Other targets for drug design
Another approach to drug development has been to identify metabolic pathways or enzymes that are specific to the parasite concerned and could be potential targets for new drugs. Thus some enzymes involved in carbohydrate metabolism, such as glyceraldehyde 3-phosphate dehydrogenase, have been identified in pathogenic trypanosomes. In addition, enzymes involved in the biosynthesis of trypanothione, a kinetoplastid-specific coenzyme and the *T. cruzi*-specific trans-sialidase are under study as potential targets for chemo-

therapy. In addition, both synthetic and natural compounds have been assayed as enzyme inhibitors.

2.4.3 *Acute phase*

Symptomatic treatment

In the majority of uncomplicated cases, symptoms usually disappear spontaneously in 4–8 weeks. During that time, it may be necessary to control various clinical manifestations with antipyretics, antiemetics, antidiarrhoeals, or electrolyte supplementation. In cases with evidence of neurological involvement, sedatives and anticonvulsants may be needed.

In patients with symptomatic acute myocarditis and manifestations of heart failure, it is necessary to prescribe diuretics and digitalis, and to restrict sodium intake. In most cases, symptoms subside in 6–8 weeks. In the rare cases of meningoencephalitis, intravenous mannitol may be necessary in addition to anticonvulsants and sedatives. In extremely severe acute cases with a high degree of myocardiopathy and for meningoencephalitis, radical treatment, such as the combination of corticoid drugs with specific parasitological treatment, could be attempted.

Etiological treatment

The acute phase of Chagas disease is characterized by the presence of parasites that are easily demonstrable in peripheral blood. Etiological treatment clears parasites from the peripheral blood and shortens the duration of the symptoms, including those of acute myocarditis and meningoencephalitis when present. If serological tests were positive, they may become negative, which indicates that the disease has been cured. This may take 6–12 months.

In uncomplicated cases and in patients with a weight of up to 40 kg, the dose of benznidazole is 7.5 mg/kg daily. In patients with body weight over 40 kg, the recommended dose is 5 mg/kg daily. Acute meningoencephalitis requires a dose of up to 25 mg/kg daily. The drug must be administered in such a way that the total daily dose is distributed in 2 or 3 doses at regular intervals during the day for 60 days.

In congenital cases, full-term neonates are treated with a daily dose of 10 mg/kg of benznidazole. Treatment must start with a dose of 5 mg/kg daily and if, after 3 days of treatment, there is neither leukopenia nor thrombocytopenia, the dose should be increased to 10 mg/kg daily.

In all cases, treatment with either benznidazole or nifurtimox should be given for 60 days. In organ transplants, infected donors should be treated for 2 weeks before the donation and recipients for 2 weeks after it. When the infection is acquired because of a laboratory accident, usually in an adult, treatment must be initiated immediately, even before the disease has been confirmed parasitologically. In these cases, the recommended dose of benznidazole is 7–10 mg/kg daily for 10 days (see also Annex 1).

2.4.4 *Chronic phase*

Symptomatic treatment

Treatment of chronic Chagas disease is aimed at alleviating symptoms and preventing complications. Heart failure is treated conventionally with sodium restriction, diuretics, and digitalis. Patients with heart damage are prone to develop cardiac arrhythmias in response to regular doses of digitalis, mainly when serum potassium is low. Beta-blockers, angiotensin-converting enzyme inhibitors, and angiotensin A_1 receptor blockers, as well as spironolactone, are also used. Tachyarrhythmias are especially resistant to most antiarrhythmic drugs and not all such drugs are well tolerated. Amiodarone has been extensively used and proved to be effective in the treatment of ventricular extrasystoles and tachycardias without interfering with cardiac performance. Patients prone to frequent episodes of sustained ventricular tachycardia — mainly with haemodynamic decompensation — and ventricular fibrillation can be treated with an automatic implantable cardiodefibrillator. In patients with symptomatic brady-cardia, high-degree sinoatrial block, or advanced or complete atrio-ventricular block, a pacemaker is indicated.

Patients predisposed to thromboembolic episodes — mainly those in whom echocardiographic studies disclose intracavitary thrombi — benefit from anticoagulant therapy.

Surgery for aneurismectomy or cavity reduction to improve haemo-dynamics has been suggested. Cardiac transplant for advanced cases is another possibility in the therapeutic spectrum of resources for the treatment of heart failure or refractory and severe cardiac arrhythmias.

The aim of the treatment of mega-oesophagus is to improve oesoph-ageal function. As in idiopathic achalasia, treatment consists of the forced dilation of the cardias with a pneumatic or hydrostatic balloon or surgery. Dilation used to be the first option and surgical procedures were reserved for cases of unsuccessful dilation or relapse. However, with the improvement in the surgical techniques used for the treatment of mega-oesophagus and the unsatisfactory long-term results obtained with dilation, the current first option for treating ectasic forms is surgery.

Apart from surgical techniques, a new approach is the injection of botulinus toxin in the lower oesophageal sphincter. This alternative and palliative treatment should be used only in selected cases. Experience with botulinus toxin is limited, but the best results following its intrasphincter injection are seen in the initial stages of the disease. An endoscopic examination should be performed before any treatment is given in order to determine whether any other associated pathological conditions are present.

Surgical treatment of megacolon is indicated in severely obstipated patients or in the presence of complications such as faecaloma, faecal impacting, or volvulus. Clinical treatment, by means of diet, laxatives, or intestinal enemas, should be provided when surgery is temporarily or definitively contraindicated for some reason.

Etiological treatment

A consensus has recently emerged that patients with chronic Chagas disease should be treated with parasiticides (*38*). This is based on the observation that the parasite can be found in chronic heart lesions and on the results of two simultaneous controlled clinical studies, carried out under the same protocol in Argentina and Brazil, of schoolchildren aged 12 years or less with positive serological tests for Chagas disease (initial chronic phase). Both clinical studies revealed that these tests were turned to negative in up to 60% of the patients after specific treatment with benznidazole in doses of 5 mg/kg daily (*35, 36*). In order to be sure that the patient is cured, the specific conventional serological test must remain negative for up to 3–5 years.

A significantly lower prevalence of heart complications and a better clinical outcome after a long follow-up of adult patients treated with parasiticidal drugs has also been reported (*37*). Hence, every patient can benefit from treatment with benznidazole, 5 mg/kg daily, or nifurtimox, 8–10 mg/kg daily, for 60 days. The total daily dose of benznidazole is given in two or three doses every 8 or 12 hours, preferably after meals. Nifurtimox is administered every 8 hours, also after meals. The treating physician should determine the age limits and the clinical suitability of this specific treatment.

Treatment of patients in the chronic phase of Chagas disease should be given only in areas where vectorial transmission has been interrupted and where it is feasible to complete the 60-day treatment under medical supervision.

In individuals with simultaneous *T. cruzi* and HIV infections, it is recommended that benznidazole, 5 mg/kg daily, should be given three times a week in order to prevent reactivation produced by immunosuppression. This prophylactic treatment is not justified in infected individuals who are receiving multidrug retroviral treatment.

2.4.5 *Assessment of cure*

An individual can be said to be cured only when a previous positive conventional serological test turns to negative. In adult patients in the chronic phase of the disease, this may take up to 10–20 years.

3. Parasitology

3.1 Taxonomy

Trypanosoma cruzi belongs to the Mastigophora subphylum of the phylum Sarcomastigophora, order Kinetoplastida, which comprises flagellar organisms with a kinetoplast, an organelle located in the cell mitochondrion which contains a fibrous network of DNA. *T. cruzi* is included in the stercorarian section, together with the group of trypanosomes whose infective stages develop in the vectors' digestive tract and contaminate the mammalian hosts through faeces. The subgenus *Schizotrypanum* has been adopted for trypanosomes that multiply in vertebrates via intracellular stages. Hence the full taxonomic name is *Trypanosoma (Schizotrypanum) cruzi* (see Fig. 1).

3.2 Isolation and maintenance of *T. cruzi* strains

A *T. cruzi* strain is defined as any parasite isolate obtained from a naturally infected insect vector, mammalian reservoir or humans. Stocks are recently isolated non-characterized strains. A strain usually consists of a genetically heterogeneous population of parasites. *T. cruzi* strains can be obtained from mammalian hosts by xenodiagnosis, haemoculture, and the direct inoculation of blood into experimental animals. Further amplification is achieved by serial passages in liquid culture medium (liver infusion-tryptose, LIT), through experimental animals, or by the infection of cultured mammalian cells. It should be pointed out that these procedures may promote the selection of a particular parasite population from the original strain. Parasite isolates can be maintained indefinitely by cryopreservation. The use of an adequate standard international code for strains and preserved parasite populations is strongly recommended (see Annex 2).

3.3 Biological characteristics

T. cruzi strains show great diversity in many biological parameters. The parasite infects a wide range of vertebrate hosts, and over 100 mammalian species have been naturally or experimentally infected

Figure 1

Classification of mammalian trypanosomes[a]

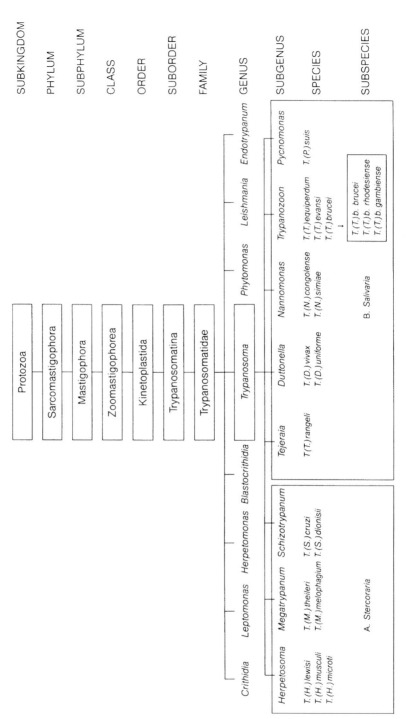

SUBKINGDOM · PHYLUM · SUBPHYLUM · CLASS · ORDER · SUBORDER · FAMILY · GENUS · SUBGENUS · SPECIES · SUBSPECIES

[a] Reproduced from WHO Technical Report Series, No. 739, 1986 (*Epidemiology and control of African trypanosomiasis: report of a WHO Expert Committee*).

with it. In experimental mice, trypomastigote blood forms may differ in morphology (slender, broad, and stout forms), and different patterns of parasitaemia may occur. Strain-dependent variations in the distribution of the intracellular amastigote forms in the tissues have been reported. Some strains display a preferential tropism for macrophages in the spleen, liver, and bone marrow, whereas others are very scarce in these organs. Variable patterns of virulence, course of parasitaemia, and mortality rates have been described (*43*). The same parasite strain may also behave differently in different lineages of mice. Experimental work in opossums indicates that some strains cause mild infection, whereas others are eliminated through immune mechanisms that are not fully understood. Molecular biology techniques have shown that, in human patients, genetically different *T. cruzi* strains may parasitize different organs.

In-vitro studies have shown differences in the invasion capability of trypomastigotes from particular strains in cultured mammalian cells. The involvement of several surface molecules of the parasite in the penetration event, such as trans-sialidase and glycoproteins of various molecular masses, has been established through biochemical techniques.

T. cruzi strains exhibit different degrees of sensitivity to chemotherapeutic agents. Natural resistance to benznidazole and nifurtimox, the two drugs widely used up to now for the treatment of Chagas disease, has been reported. This should be kept in mind whenever new drugs are tested.

3.4 Genetic characteristics

Considerable advances have been made in the understanding of the genetics of *T. cruzi* and of the processes involved in the control of gene expression. Many genes coding for structural components, metabolic enzymes, molecules involved in penetration, and immunodominant antigens have been cloned and sequenced. Recombinant proteins bearing immunodominant domains have been expressed and used as reagents for serodiagnosis. The development of cloning vectors for transfection studies has made it possible to knock out some genes and to super-express others in order to elucidate their role in the biology of the parasite.

Genetic molecular markers of *T. cruzi* have been sought in an effort to correlate the different strains with their biological properties, clinical manifestations, and epidemiological characteristics. Early studies of population genetics revealed a substantial isozymic variability among isolates of *T. cruzi*, defining three major groups or zymodemes named Z1, Z2, and Z3 (*44*). Z2 was associated with the domestic transmission cycle, whereas Z1 and Z3 were predominant in the sylvatic cycle. Further analysis of 15 gene loci of isoenzymes disclosed a greater heterogeneity determining the distribution of 121 *T. cruzi* isolates from the American continent into 43 zymodemes that could not be grouped by the authors into a few natural clusters. The main conclusion of these studies was that the population structure of *T. cruzi* is clonal rather than sexual and, as a consequence, the present genetic biological variability is the result of the independent evolution of clonal lines (*45*). In Argentina, 12 zymodeme groups were reported, of which six were isolated from humans but only two were widely distributed in the endemic areas. One of these zymodemes was closely associated with the incidence of acute symptomatic infection and with chronic cardiopathy.

Restriction-fragment-length polymorphism in kinetoplast DNA (kDNA) of *T. cruzi* showed highly heterogeneous patterns in parasite isolates defining several groups known as schizodemes (*46*). Nuclear DNA fingerprinting and karyotyping studies have confirmed the genetic complexity of *T. cruzi* populations.

In contrast to the wide polymorphism of isoenzymes and restriction fragments of kDNA, analysis of the ribosomal RNA (rRNA) gene and intergenic sequences showed dimorphism among parasite strains. PCR amplification of a specific region of the 24S alpha rRNA gene produced fragments of 125 bp and 110 bp which defined two principal groups of strains. These groups were confirmed by randomly amplified polymorphic DNA (RAPD) analysis of 50–60 polymorphic loci (*47, 48*). The existence of the two groups of strains was also verified by detailed isoenzyme data, riboprinting analysis, and biological behaviour in mice (biodemes).

A proposed standardization of the nomenclature of the two principal groups of strains of *T. cruzi* is shown in Box 1 (*49*).

Box 1

Standardization of the nomenclature of the two principal groups of strains of *Trypanosoma cruzi*

***T. cruzi* I** = equivalent to zymodeme 1 (*44*); lineage 2 (*47*); group 1 or discrete taxonomic unit (DTU) 1 (*45*); type III (*43*); ribodeme II/III (*50*)

***T. cruzi* II** = equivalent to zymodeme 2 (*44*); zymodeme A (*51*); lineage 1 (*47*); group 2 or DTU 2 (*45*); type II (*43*); ribodeme I (*50*)

According to the group equivalences shown in Box 1, rapid PCR methods for strain typing will be preferable to zymodeme typing, a procedure that requires considerable amounts of parasite cells and may promote the selection of a particular population of the original strain.

The epidemiological distribution of the two groups of strains has been investigated. *T. cruzi* isolates were obtained from mammalian reservoirs, humans, and triatomines from several regions of Bolivia, Brazil, and Colombia, and were typed by PCR as belonging to *T. cruzi* groups I and II. There is evidence of a strong association of *T. cruzi* II with the domestic cycle, while *T. cruzi* I was preferentially encountered in the sylvatic environment (*52*). Since all parasites isolated from seropositive individuals from endemic regions belong to *T. cruzi* II, it is suggested that this group has properties that favour human infections and promote higher parasitaemia. On the other hand, in Amazonas, *T. cruzi* I was isolated from wild triatomines but from only a very small number of seropositive people with low parasitaemia and the indeterminate form of Chagas disease (*52*).

The presence of two major *T. cruzi* populations designated clone 20 (*T. cruzi* I) and clone 39 (*T. cruzi* II) was reported in an endemic area of Bolivia. It was shown that clone 39 was more frequent in chagasic children whereas, with *Triatoma infestans*, both clones 20 and 39 were found with comparable frequencies. These observations suggest that the immune system of young patients may control the infection caused by *T. cruzi* I (*53*). A similar situation may occur in areas of high endemicity in Chile, where clone 39 is the most prevalent in congenital cases.

3.5 The parasite genome and the *T. cruzi* genome project

The *T. cruzi* genome project was launched by the UNDP/World Bank/WHO Special Programme for Research and Training in Tropical Diseases (TDR) in 1994 and was implemented by a number of research groups in Europe, South America, and the United States of America. The results obtained so far are summarized below (*54–57*):

- The biological characteristics of the CL Brener clone (group *T. cruzi* II), chosen as the reference organism of the project, have been established.
- It was estimated that the CL Brener haploid genome has approximately 40–50 Mbp and is distributed in 30–40 chromosomes.
- Genomic libraries have been constructed in different vectors.
- cDNA libraries have been obtained from messenger RNA from epimastigote forms of CL Brener.

- Random sequencing of cDNA clones yielded almost 11 000 sequences (called expression sequence tags). Approximately 15 000 sequences (called genomic sequence surveys) have been obtained from clones of genomic libraries. Both types of sequences are deposited in public databases. It is estimated that approximately 20% of the parasite genome is known.
- Gene discovery was approached through comparison of the sequences generated in the project with gene and protein sequences of other organisms deposited in databases. It was concluded that 40% of the sequences show similarities with genes corresponding to enzymes of metabolic pathways, signal transduction, structural proteins, etc. On the other hand, 60% of the sequences have no homology with previously reported genes and may therefore constitute *T. cruzi*-specific genes.

Additional information on the project is accessible at the web site http://www.dbbm.fiocruz.br/TcruziDB/index.html.

It is hoped that the *T. cruzi* genome project will serve to identify new targets for drug development and increase the understanding both of the host–parasite relationship and of the mechanisms involved in pathogenesis.

4. Vectors

4.1 Taxonomy

The vectors of *T. cruzi* are insects belonging to the order Hemiptera, family Reduviidae and subfamily Triatominae. Currently, over 130 species are known, belonging to five tribes (Alberproseniini, Bolboderini, Cavernicolini, Rhodniini, and Triatomini) and 16 genera (*Alberprosenia*, Martínez & Carcavallo, 1977; *Bolbodera*, Valdés, 1910; *Belminus*, Stål, 1859; *Microtriatoma*, Prosen & Martínez, 1952; *Parabelminus*, Lent, 1943; *Cavernicola*, Barber, 1937; *Torrealbaia*, Carcavallo, Jurberg & Lent, 1998; *Psammolestes*, Bergroth, 1911; *Rhodnius*, Stål, 1859; *Dipetalogaster*, Usinger, 1939; *Eratyrus*, Stål, 1859; *Hermanlentia*, Jurberg & Galvão, 1997; *Mepraia*, Mazza, Gajardo & Jörg, 1940; *Panstrongylus*, Berg, 1879; *Paratriatoma*, Barber, 1938; and *Triatoma*, Laporte, 1832). However, only a few species of three genera, namely *Triatoma*, *Rhodnius*, and *Panstrongylus*, are important vectors of *T. cruzi* between domestic animals and humans in endemic areas. All three genera are widely distributed in the Americas, from Mexico to Argentina and Chile. Wild Triatominae species have a still wider distribution, from the north of the USA to the Patagonian region in the south (*58, 59*).

Most species of Triatominae live in natural habitats in contact with birds, mammals, and reptiles in different ecosystems. Some species can survive only within a narrow range of temperatures (e.g. *Belminus laportei* and *Triatoma dispar* — stenothermic species), and humidity (e.g. *Dipetalogaster maxima, Triatoma breyeri*, and *Belminus pittieri* — stenohydric species). Others can tolerate a broad range of climatic conditions (e.g. *Panstrongylus geniculatus, Triatoma infestans*, and *Mepraia spinolai* — eurithermic species). Others Triatominae require specific sources of food, e.g. *Cavernicola pilosa*, which feeds on bats, and *Triatoma protracta*, which feeds on spiny rats of the genus *Neotoma*; these are stenophagous species. Other — euriphagous — species have no special feeding preferences; these include *Triatoma guasayana, T. sanguisuga*, and *T. sordida* (*60*).

4.2 Geographical distribution

Most species are found between the parallels 45°S and 40°N, and at altitudes up to 1500 metres above sea level. They are prevalent in areas between the tropics. However, some species are found in temperate regions with cold winters, e.g. *T. patagonica* and *T. infestans*, which are common in Argentine Patagonia, or *T. sanguisuga*, found in the USA in Indiana and Maryland. This can be explained by the microclimatic conditions of the ecotopes, which are generally warmer than the external environment (*59*).

The species epidemiologically linked to human Chagas disease are those that have adapted to the human environment. The geographical distribution of the most important vectors of the disease in the Americas before the implementation of vector-control programmes was as follows:

- *Triatoma infestans*
  - Argentina, except the province of Santa Cruz
  - Bolivia (Beni, Chuquisaca, Cochabamba, La Paz, Potosí, Santa Cruz, Tarija)
  - Brazil (states of Alagoas, Bahia, Goiás, Mato Grosso, Mato Grosso do Sul, Minas Gerais, Paraíba, Paraná, Pernambuco, Piauí, Rio de Janeiro, Rio Grande do Sul, São Paulo, Sergipe, Tocantins)
  - Chile (Regions I–VI and the metropolitan Santiago area)
  - Paraguay (Alto Paraguay, Boquerón, Caaguazú, Caazapá, Central, Chaco, Concepción, Cordillera, Guairá, Misiones, Nueva Asunción, Paraguarí, Presidente Hayes, San Pedro)
  - Peru (Arequipa, Ica, Moquegua, Tacna)
  - Uruguay.

- *Rhodnius prolixus*
  — Colombia (Antioquia, Arauca, Boyacá, Caquetá, Casanare, César, Cundinamarca, Guajira, Huila, Magdalena, Meta, Norte de Santander, Putumayo, Santander, Tolima, Vichada)
  — El Salvador
  — Guatemala (in five of the 22 departments)
  — Honduras (in 11 of the 18 departments)
  — Mexico (Chiapas, Oaxaca)
  — Nicaragua
  — Venezuela (Aragua, Carabobo, Cojedes, Miranda, Portuguesa, Yaracuy).

- *Triatoma dimidiata*
  — Belize
  — Colombia
  — Costa Rica
  — Ecuador
  — El Salvador
  — Guatemala
  — Honduras (in 16 of the 18 departments)
  — Mexico (Campeche, Chiapas, Guerrero, Jalisco, Nayarit, Oaxaca, Puebla, Quintana Róo, San Luis Potosi, Tabasco, Veracruz, Yucatan)
  — Nicaragua
  — Panama
  — Peru (Tumbes)
  — Venezuela.

- *Panstrongylus megistus*
  — Argentina (Corrientes, Jujuy, Misiones, Salta)
  — Brazil (Alagoas, Bahia, Ceará, Espirito Santo, Goiás, Maranhão, Mato Grosso, Mato Grosso do Sul, Minas Gerais, Pará, Paraíba, Paraná, Pernambuco, Piauí, Rio de Janeiro, Rio Grande del Norte, Rio Grande do Sul, Santa Catarina, São Paulo, Sergipe)
  — Paraguay (Amambay, Cordillera)
  — Uruguay.

- *Triatoma brasiliensis*
  — Brazil (widespread in all the semi-arid north-east of the country — Alagoas, Bahia, Ceará, Maranhão, Paraíba, Piauí, Rio Grande del Norte, Sergipe, Tocantins — and the north of Minas Gerais).

At present, the geographical distribution of the domiciliated species has been significantly reduced by the activities of the control programmes in some countries. This is true for *T. infestans* in Brazil, Chile, and Uruguay and in some areas of Argentina, and for *R. prolixus* in Venezuela and in some areas of Honduras and Nicaragua (see Fig. 2, which also shows the distribution of *T. dimidiata*).

4.3 Biology

After eclosion, the insects of the subfamily Triatominae pass through five nymphal instars before reaching the adult stage. During all these phases they are generally haematophagous. Under laboratory conditions, triatomine development is completed in about six months, varying according to the species. Generally, the time taken is longer in the natural environment. A female *T. infestans* can lay up to 600 eggs during her lifetime of a year and a half. The mean duration of egg incubation is 18–20 days. Adult insects may copulate several times during their lives, thus increasing genetic variability.

Triatomines can fast for periods of up to 200 days but to develop they must have a blood meal. They are normally active at night. *T. infestans* has two peaks of activity, one at dusk and the other at dawn, corresponding to searching for food and for hiding places to rest, respectively. Activity is controlled by light and temperature. Other species reveal interesting variations, e.g. in *T. brasiliensis*, which is adapted to dry environments with high temperatures and abundant light, peak activity occurs at the end of the day, in synchronization with the nocturnal habits of the rodents that are its natural hosts.

The fact that triatomines are obligatory blood-feeders explains the strict relationship between the insects and their feeding sources which markedly affects their biology and behaviour. Some species are highly adapted to a single host, and are able to survive only in the microhabitat occupied by this particular host. This group includes *Psammolestes*, which colonizes the nests of birds of the family Furnariidae. Under laboratory conditions, its nymphs rarely reach the adult phase, making it difficult to maintain for more than one generation. *T. infestans* can be considered to be highly adapted to the domestic environment; it has little chance of survival in the wild, except in its area of origin in Bolivia, where it forms small colonies in association with wild rodents and lizards. Other species, such as *P. geniculatus*, *P. megistus*, *T. brasiliensis*, and *T. dimidiata*, are more eclectic, and can adapt more easily to different habitats.

Genetic studies have demonstrated a correlation between adaptation to different ecotopes and genetic variability. In contrast, specificity of

Figure 2
Current geographical distribution of the three triatomine vector species of major epidemiological importance in Chagas disease

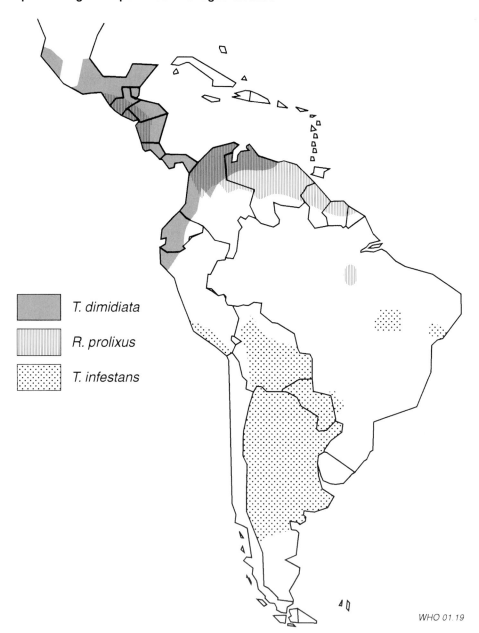

T. dimidiata

R. prolixus

T. infestans

WHO 01.19

ecotopes is associated with genetic simplification: species that are more vulnerable to environmental changes may disappear in situations of ecological imbalance, or become more susceptible to control measures. This is seen with *T. infestans* in South America and *R. prolixus* in Central America and northern South America. However, *T. infestans* has developed a biological mechanism to compensate for such genetic simplification, namely polyandric fertilization, in which a female copulates successively with several males.

Competition for food may stimulate the adults to search for new habitats, and to leave sylvatic ecotopes in the so-called "infestation period". For *P. megistus*, *T. dimidiata*, and *T. brasiliensis*, this period corresponds to the rainy months; for *T. sordida*, it occurs at the beginning of the dry season.

Unfavourable environmental changes cause triatomines to move to man-made habitats, which are highly stable and offer a variety of hiding places and an abundance of food throughout the year. Thanks to this environmental stability, domiciliary populations of triatomines may reach much higher densities than those seen in sylvatic habitats.

For the majority of species, the size of the colony of triatomines associated with humans is an important factor in the transmission of Chagas disease. The size of the colony, in turn, depends on the number of hosts and the degree of triatomine–host adaptation, which permits the triatomine to obtain the blood necessary for the completion of its life cycle in the shortest period. In one study, *T. infestans* was able to obtain a full blood meal from non-anaesthetized mice in 4 hours — the same time as that required to feed on anaesthetized animals; *R. prolixus*, however, ingested only 46.7% of the weight of blood obtained by insects in a control group during the same period (*61*). These observations can be explained by the greater irritation caused by the bite of *R. prolixus*, which makes the host uncomfortable and interferes with the process of blood feeding. In addition, some species may possess a more rapid suction mechanism. *T. infestans* feeds more rapidly than *T. brasiliensis* and *T. pseudomaculata*, whatever the blood source.

The saliva of triatomines is of great importance in feeding. It is known that the salivary proteins differ from one species to another. Species whose bites are more painful or cause strong allergic reactions, such as *P. geniculatus*, *T. protracta*, *T. rubida*, and *T. rubrofasciata*, are less likely to colonize human dwellings.

Most species of triatomines have exclusively sylvatic habits, and may be found, for example, under the bark of dead trees, in tree hollows, in the shelters of opossums, bats, rodents, etc., in piles of rocks, in the leaves of various plants such as palms and bromeliads, in birds' nests, and in burrows made by animals such as armadillos. In the absence of a warm-blooded feeding source, some triatomines can also feed on reptiles and amphibians. Certain species, such as *T. rubrovaria*, have preserved their ancestral predatory habits and can feed on the larvae of other insects.

Triatomines that colonize houses permanently and are markedly anthropophilic are considered to be of primary epidemiological importance. They are found in cracks in walls, under loose plaster and packing cases, and behind pictures and wall ornaments. Triatomines of secondary importance can produce small, more transitory, intra-domiciliary colonies, especially in the absence of primary vectors. They show different degrees of anthropophily, but are well adapted to artificial ecotopes.

The distribution of triatomines is typically focal, and population density is conditioned by the availability of food. Ecotopes are considered to be stable when the feeding source is always present and hiding places are permanent, permitting the development of larger colonies, as occurs with *R. neglectus* in various palm trees. In this habitat, the majority of the feeding sources are birds. Even when these migrate, other vertebrates, including cold-blooded animals, can serve as blood meal sources for the triatomines. In spite of fluctuations in *R. neglectus* populations throughout the year, colonies do not disappear during the months when food is scarce.

Until recently, Amazonia was considered to be outside the risk area for triatomine domiciliation. However, 18 species of triatomines are known to occur in the Amazon basin, which is now at risk of domiciliation mainly because of poorly planned colonization of the region by immigrants from other areas, and uncontrolled deforestation. The behaviour of *R. brethesi* is especially noteworthy; this species lives in *piaçava* palms, emerging to attack palm-nut collectors. The presence of *P. geniculatus*, widely distributed in Brazil and other countries, in the artificial environment is so far restricted to occasional invasions by flying adults.

4.4 Ecology and behaviour of triatomines

All species of triatomines are adapted to live in a particular environment. A classification based on vector habitat, which has important implications for control and includes the characteristics of the most important species, has been adopted here (*62*).

4.4.1 *Species strictly domiciliated or exceptionally found in wild ecotopes*

Triatoma infestans and *T. rubrofasciata* are among the species that are strictly domiciliated or, exceptionally, found in wild ecotopes. *T. infestans* is a native of Bolivia, the only country where its existence in the sylvatic environment has been proven. In its natural habitat, it lives in association with rodents, under piles of rocks. Adapted since the pre-Columbian period to human dwellings, it has been dispersed passively to Argentina, Brazil, Chile, Paraguay, southern Peru, and Uruguay. Predominantly domiciliar, *T. infestans* is considered to be the most important triatomine species in all the countries where it has been found. Closely associated with human beings and domestic animals in their dispersion, populations with very simplified genetic characteristics have been selected, resulting in low variability and an inability to adapt to changing environments. This extreme adaptation to human dwellings has made *T. infestans* the most important vector of human Chagas disease, but has also resulted in greater genetic fragility, making possible its complete elimination in most of the areas in which it occurs.

T. rubrofasciata can be considered to be the only strictly domiciliated triatomine. It is found in coastal regions throughout the neotropics, intimately associated with the domestic rat (*Rattus rattus*) and transmitting *Trypanosoma conorhini*.

4.4.2 *Species found in both domestic and wild ecotopes, with frequent domiciliated colonies*

These include *Panstrongylus megistus*, *Rhodnius pallescens*, *R. prolixus*, *Triatoma barberi*, *T. brasiliensis*, *T. dimidiata*, *T. guasayana*, *T. longipennis*, *T. maculata*, *T. phyllosoma*, *T. pseudomaculata*, and *T. sordida*. *R. prolixus* is undoubtedly the most important of these species, since it is the principal vector of Chagas disease in Central America, Colombia, and Venezuela. It has been reported in the wild in palms and the nests of herons, from which it could colonize houses by passive or active transport. Its sylvatic origin remains doubtful because of the lack of morphometric and isoenzyme differentiation between *Rhodnius* found in Venezuelan palm trees (identified as *R. robustus*) and the typical *R. prolixus* found inside houses. It is captured mainly in the straw roofs of houses, where it reaches very high densities. Humidity appears to be an essential factor in its development, particularly with regard to the eclosion of the eggs. Recent genetic studies support the hypothesis of the passive introduction of this species in Central America, where it is found only inside houses.

In this area, it is considered to be responsible for most *T. cruzi* vectorial transmission.

T. sordida is the species most often captured in Brazil since the 1980s, particularly in the peridomestic environment. It is able to adapt to highly unstable environments, and evidence of its biological potential is provided by colonies close to houses. Despite being markedly ornithophilic, it may also colonize houses. It is found mainly under the bark of dry or dead trees, where colonies consist of a few individuals, the majority without blood in the digestive tube, demonstrating the sporadic availability of feeding sources in these ecotopes.

P. megistus inhabits sparse woods or gallery forests, but is of epidemiological importance in those regions where it is sometimes the only triatomine found in houses.

T. brasiliensis is the main representative of the autochthonous triatomines of the semi-arid interplateau depressions that constitute the dominant landscape of north-east Brazil. It is found in the sylvatic environment under large piles of rocks, and is associated with rodents, whose burrows provide a year-round stable environment and permit the development of large colonies, sometimes close to houses. Highly active, these insects can be observed during the day emerging from their hiding places among the piles of rocks to attack their hosts, exposing themselves to intense sunlight and high temperatures. Twelve months after the treatment of infested houses with pyrethroids, original populations have been known to be replaced by individuals that survive spraying and adults that invade houses by flying.

T. pseudomaculata, has its natural ecotopes under bark, in the hollows of dead dry trees, and in birds' nests. Although little is known about the dispersal of *T. pseudomaculata*, passive transport in firewood must certainly play a role in the introduction of this triatomine into the artificial environment. Large colonies may be formed in the peridomestic environment, but in general this species is poorly adapted to living in houses.

T. dimidiata also has a wide geographical distribution (from northern South America to Central America and Mexico) and is of great epidemiological importance. Its natural ecotopes include the burrows of opossums (in which it is responsible for high rates of *T. cruzi* infection), the trunks of trees, and piles of rocks. Two important aspects of its ecology distinguish this species from the majority of triatomines: the frequency with which it colonizes urban areas and its capacity to transmit *T. cruzi* to humans at very low densities. It is also unusual in its association with the floors of houses, where it covers itself with dust as camouflage. Despite its passive introduction into houses from woods, knowledge of its population dynamics is limited.

R. pallescens is the main vector in Panama, where it occurs in palms, feeding on opossums, anteaters, sloths, rodents, birds, and, more rarely, lizards. In houses, it frequently feeds on humans, and in the peridomestic environment on pigeons and chickens.

T. barberi has a wide distribution in Mexico, where it colonizes houses and the peridomestic environment and shows very aggressive behaviour, biting both during the day and at night.

4.4.3 *Species mainly wild, but sometimes captured in the domestic environment*

These include *Panstrongylus lutzi, Rhodnius ecuadoriensis, R. nasutus, R. neglectus, R. pictipes, Triatoma lecticularia, T. nitida, T. rubrovaria,* and *T. vitticeps.*

T. rubrovaria is the predominant species in the prairies of southern Brazil. In recent years, it has been increasingly found in artificial environments, including houses. In Uruguay, it is encountered among piles of rocks, sometimes very close to houses, in close association with cockroaches and other insects on which it feeds. Furthermore, *T. vitticeps* and *P. lutzi* have been found to be highly infected with *T. cruzi,* which emphasizes the need for strict surveillance of these species.

4.4.4 *Wild species, with adults seldom found in dwellings*

These include *Microtriatoma trinidadensis, Panstrongylus rufotuberculatus, Triatoma breyeri, T. carrioni, T. circummaculata, T. guazu, T. jurbergi, T. mazzotti, T. melanocephala, T. pallidipennis, T. patagonica, T. platensis, T. protracta, T. ryckmani, T. sanguisuga,* and *T. tibiamaculata.*

4.4.5 *Species found only in wild ecotopes*

These include *Alberprosenia* spp., *Belminus* spp., *Bolbodera scabrosa, Cavernicola* spp., *Hermanlentia matsunoi, Mepraia* spp., *Parabelminus* spp., *Paratriatoma hirsuta, Torrealbaia martinez,* and many species of the genus *Triatoma.*

4.5 Climatic factors and dispersion and adaptation of triatomines

In 1913, it was found that warming shortens the embryonic period of *T. infestans.* Further work showed that, in areas with high temperatures, *T. infestans* has two generations per year, while in temperate or cold areas, it has only one generation during the same period. Shorter life cycles were also observed in colonies of three species of the genus *Triatoma* kept permanently at 27–28 °C compared with colonies reared outdoors at variable temperatures, including cold weather during winter. Temperature affects the hatching time of the eggs, the time required to complete the life cycle, the biting rate or feeding frequency, the metabolism, and seasonality. Low relative humidity can increase the feeding frequency because of dehydration.

The influence of microclimatic conditions on habitats has been studied in Argentina and Venezuela. The temperature inside the palm tree *Attalea butyraceae* was usually constant at 22–23 °C, while in the external environment it varied from 16 °C to 30 °C. Relative humidity was also always high inside the palm tree, but varied from 40 to 95 % on the external leaves. Triatomines move around inside the tree so as to obtain the best conditions of temperature and humidity.

Recent observations on climate change, especially on global warming and the El Niño Southern Oscillation (ENSO), have shown that higher temperatures may increase the geographical distribution of vectors and the altitude at which they can survive. This is particularly important for wild species with a tendency to invade human habitats. Lower humidity, while possibly extending their geographical distribution and increasing their population density, can adversely affect their life cycles in dry tropical and subtropical environments and arid areas. If the indoor temperature increases, vector species in the domestic environment can develop shorter life cycles and greater population densities. However, for domiciliated species, human activities such as replastering walls and applying chemical agents may be more significant than climatic conditions in determining the vector population density.

4.5.1 *Sylvatic ecotopes and the domiciliation process*

Triatomines were originally sylvatic but some species have gradually become domiciliated. Sylvatic populations (adults and nymphs) can be found in a great variety of ecotopes. Anthropic environmental modifications have led to the disappearance of the natural foci, leading to the domiciliation of triatomines.

The nature and quality of buildings, as well as housing conditions (including the storage of goods and belongings inside and around the house) are important determinants of the colonization of human dwellings by triatomines. Domiciliary and peridomestic habitats may create favourable microhabitats and provide protection from predators. Other factors include the abundant blood supply offered by humans as well as the protection found by the vector on the surfaces of mud walls.

Domiciliary habitats related to house construction include cracks and crevices in mud or concrete walls, the junctions between adobe or concrete bricks, spaces between pieces of wood or cane, roofs made of palm trees, and earthen floors. Other factors that favour bug infestation include the storage of harvested crops in the house, collections of adobe blocks in indoor passages and corridors, and piles of sticks in the house.

The presence of animals in the house, the type of construction of any outbuildings (for storage or for animals), and the closeness of such outbuildings to the house also have an important influence on the presence of vectors and the transmission of the parasite.

4.5.2 *The changes associated with domiciliation*

The domiciliation of triatomines is the main factor in increasing the risk of *T. cruzi* transmission to humans. Some techniques, e.g. multilocus enzyme electrophoresis (MLEE), DNA methods, or morphometrics, can help in elucidating the genetic and phenotypic changes associated with domiciliation. These techniques have shown that the process is usually associated with major migrations, the reduction of genetic repertoire, and increasing developmental instability, making the insect a more efficient vector as well as a more vulnerable target of control measures.

Since only some of the sylvatic genotypes may be successful in establishing durable domestic colonies, some restriction of genetic variability is assumed to occur during the early stages of the domiciliation process. The dispersion of the insect becomes dependent on its host and may be boosted by passive transport. The insect is likely to be transported by humans (or domestic animals) over large distances, beyond the current range of its ecological constraints. As a consequence of both isolation from the original sylvatic foci and founder effects in the new areas of colonization, a further loss of genetic variability is to be expected. As long as this geographical expansion continues, domiciliation becomes a more exclusive habit, and some populations with high levels of inbreeding may show external evidence of developmental instability, such as increased fluctuating asymmetry or unilateral morphological monstrosity. Size and sexual dimorphism may also be reduced.

Such populations, like most domestic *T. infestans* or *R. prolixus* populations, should be more vulnerable to control measures. However, the dramatic geographical spread apparently associated with domiciliation is of concern, and reinforces the need for careful entomological surveillance of those triatomines that currently exhibit trends towards it, e.g. *T. brasiliensis*, *T. dimidiata*, and *T. nitida*.

4.6 Population genetics

Population genetics applies specifically to natural populations of an organism. The word "population" refers to individuals of the same species, forming distinct groups on the basis of geographical, ecological, behavioural, and/or epidemiological criteria. The main epidemiological applications of population genetics in triatomines are those concerned with systematics and studies of population structure.

Population genetics focuses on genes, DNA fragments, or any trait considered to be a Mendelian factor, and their frequencies in various populations. Relevant techniques include the traditional MLEE and the more recent DNA methods. Analytical methods currently rely on certain probabilistic models defining genetic equilibrium. They delineate the expected features of genetic variability (heterozygosity) as well as of gene frequencies — or the frequency of DNA fragments — within and among populations. When applied to epidemiological problems, however, such theoretical approaches have at least two main drawbacks. First, they are based on population models, which are not very realistic. Second, the gene flow that can be estimated from gene frequencies is not necessarily taking place at the time of the study; it might have occurred in the past, even in the recent past, and might have been exhausted.

From an epidemiological point of view, the main question is not whether changes have occurred in the past, but whether they are occurring now. For instance, are sylvatic *T. infestans* in Cochabamba able to reinvade houses following insecticide treatment? What is important is not whether the sylvatic foci concerned were connected to human dwellings in the past, but whether they are now. To answer such questions, mark–recapture techniques could be used. However, this approach is generally appropriate only for flying adults, while in triatomines the main mode of dispersion seems to be the passive transportation of juvenile stages of species rarely associated with humans.

For all these reasons, various indirect methods and techniques have been used for studying population structure, including cytogenetics and cytometry, as well as traditional and geometric morphometrics.

4.7 Epidemiological application of the new tools

The two areas of population genetics that may be of epidemiological relevance are systematics and population structure studies.

4.7.1 *Systematics*

Systematics is the oldest and best known application of population genetics in medical entomology, where it is used to identify the correct species and target for insecticide control. For the triatomines, the main techniques that have been used for distinguishing between similar taxa include cytogenetics, MLEE, and DNA methods.

Colombia has provided the right conditions for testing this methodology since *R. prolixus*, which is common in this country (see p. 42), can be both domiciliated and wild. Indeed, evidence suggests the existence of two *Rhodnius* species. The sylvatic population was recently described as *Rhodnius colombiensis* (*63*). When DNA from domiciliated and wild *Rhodnius* individuals was amplified by PCR using rDNA universal primers, two bands were found, but the amplification of the second band was sometimes low or absent. This result suggests that the wild and domiciliated populations of *Rhodnius* have at least two distinct forms of rDNA, which differ from each other in size, and shows that PCR amplification can differentiate between sylvatic and domiciliated populations of *R. prolixus*. The differences are consistent with a model in which molecular drive rapidly gives rise to unique spacer patterns in populations and then drives them to high frequencies. Such patterns are consistent with what might be expected for population differentiation resulting from genetic drift and restricted gene flow. They are also consistent with the low gene flow between domiciliated and wild *Rhodnius* populations found using RAPD analysis.

Recently applied DNA-based methods, such as sequencing, have initially focused on evolutionary genetics, but the taxonomic problems in the reliable identification of subspecies or related species have also been addressed. These approaches have recently confirmed the genetic proximity of *T. melanosoma* and *T. infestans* and the evolutionary divergence between *R. robustus* and *R. prolixus*. Both findings are epidemiologically important. The first shows the phenotypic plasticity of *T. infestans*, which is able to adapt to new ecotopes such as houses or trees; the second allows more specific targeting of *R. prolixus* in insecticide campaigns.

4.7.2 *Population structure*

Exchanges of individuals between geographical populations of the vector are rare or accidental (poor gene flow). Such populations have therefore become isolated. A control campaign may thus be conducted without great risk of reinvasion from untreated areas. When based on gene frequencies, such a conclusion relies on the recognition of certain population models. If genetic differences are estimated in the absence of precise knowledge of gene frequencies, the relevant result is a significant difference between two populations. Indeed, such differences indicate that migrations are unlikely.

An intraspecific study of cytogenetic variation describing population structure was carried out on the populations of *T. infestans* in Uruguay (*64*). Two distinct populations were found, separated by the Rio Negro and differing in their epidemiological characteristics.

The reduction in genetic variability has important consequences for control programmes. Since a reduced gene pool also implies that selection for new attributes, such as resistance to insecticides, will be less likely, and since the dispersal capacity of *R. prolixus* is very low, the probability of reinfestation by wild populations should also be low. The application of PCR to insects captured 2 years after a house-spraying programme was carried out indicated that, as shown by the amplification pattern, all the insects were domiciliated. In terms of vectorial transmission, therefore, wild populations of *R. prolixus* seem to be unimportant as possible vectors of Chagas disease in Colombia.

4.7.3 *Population movements and reinfestation*

The control of Chagas disease vectors relies primarily on the spraying of infested dwellings with pyrethroid insecticides. After the initial intervention, however, it is important to continue entomological surveillance so that any new infestations can be selectively re-treated. The reappearance of domestic vectors might be due to population movements of the bugs, in which case the nearest and most probable source would be the neighbouring foci or in some cases the local sylvatic foci. On the other hand, reinfestation might have been caused by individuals that survived the initial insecticide treatment. These two hypotheses have been explored under field conditions by means of cytogenetics, MLEE, and morphometric comparisons.

The karyotype, as defined by heterochromatic variation, was the same in both reinfesting and previously treated populations, while it was consistently different from that of neighbouring populations (*65*). This strongly suggested that reinfesting insects were residual populations not reached by previous insecticide spraying.

Simple morphometric comparisons between reinfesting insects and those present at the same place and surrounding areas before insecticide application also seem able to help in distinguishing between residual populations and reinvasion from other foci. This has been demonstrated in a village in Bolivia infested with domestic *T. infestans* and surrounded by sylvatic foci of the same species (*66*). Infestation by *T. infestans* having morphometric characteristics similar to those of the domestic insects was detected 10 months after spraying, supporting the hypothesis that few, if any, insects migrated from sylvatic to domestic ecotopes. When isoenzymes and morphometrics were used in combination to study reinfestation by *T. infestans* in houses following insecticide application, both techniques suggested that reinvasion was the most probable explanation.

4.7.4 *Historical population movements*

If the history of past population movements of the vector is known, this has two important epidemiological consequences. First, in peripheral regions where colonization is recent, control is more likely to be successful; these regions are generally free of sylvatic foci. Second, increased surveillance may be undertaken at the centre of the geographical dispersion, since it is here that there is a high probability of finding sylvatic foci and a relatively higher risk of reinfestation. It has been possible to identify such a history of past population movements by using genetic markers in two vectors, *T. infestans* and *R. prolixus*.

It is thought that *T. infestans* spread within the Andean area during the time of the Inca empire, then invaded the lowlands from Argentina to Brazil, Paraguay, and Uruguay after the Spanish conquest. Cytometric techniques show that, in the migration process, the genome of *T. infestans* decreased to about 40% of its initial size (*67*).

In Central America, the mean number of bands by primer (b/p) was half that found in South America, which might reflect a reduction in genome size. The same specimens were more alike in Central America than in South America, also suggesting a reduction in genetic variability. These observations supported a South American origin of *R. prolixus*, and its recent invasion of Central America.

Insects from Central America (Guatemala and Honduras) were more alike than those in Colombia. They also showed a significant decrease in the number of b/p, from 12 b/p in Colombia to 7.5 and 5.9 b/p in Guatemala and Honduras, respectively. These data also tend to support the hypothesis of a South American origin of *R. prolixus*.

5. Natural reservoirs

Originally, Chagas disease was a zoonosis that involved numerous sylvatic triatomines and mammals in natural foci from which humans and domestic animals were absent. As a result of human–vector contact in rural areas and changes in the natural biotopes, the disease has spread to peridomestic and domestic sites.

The natural reservoirs of *T. cruzi* are those mammals — domestic, synanthropic, and wild — including humans, that are naturally infected by the parasite. Such reservoirs play an important part in the maintenance of, and interaction between, the domestic and wild cycles of Chagas disease.

A list of sylvatic and domestic or peridomestic animal reservoir hosts of *T. cruzi* and their geographical distribution in the Americas is given in Annex 3.

5.1 Domestic and synanthropic reservoirs

Humans are the most important domestic reservoir of *T. cruzi* in the domestic cycle. Data from precipitin tests, using antisera against mammals, birds, reptiles, and amphibians, and carried out on the intestinal content of triatomines in Brazil, Chile, Costa Rica, and Venezuela, showed overall feeding rates of 50.5–91.0% for humans, 46.3–80.8% for dogs, 0.1–8.8% for cats, and 5.9–15.2% for chickens. The life expectancy of humans of more than 60 years, and the parasitaemia that may remain positive for more than 40 years indicate that humans constitute the most important reservoir (*68*). However, dogs and cats, with an average life span of 7 years, play a significant part in the dynamics of transmission in the human environment. Moreover, xenodiagnosis and/or serology indicates that a large number of domestic and synanthropic mammals in North, Central, and South America are naturally infected by the parasite. These mammals include goats, sheep, alpacas, pigs, rabbits, guinea-pigs, rats, and mice.

The proportion of *T. cruzi*-infected reservoirs will vary with the local epidemiological situation and will depend on the density of triatomines and the proportion infected in the household or geographical unit. The circulation of the parasite in the domestic cycle is dynamic, and reservoirs become infected at an early age through contact with infected triatomines.

Higher percentages of infection by *T. cruzi* in dogs and cats, which eventually exceed those found in humans, are observed in zones where *T. infestans* and other vectors present in high densities constitute the main or the only domiciliary vector.

The highly efficient transmission of *T. cruzi*, the close trophic association with *T. infestans*, the age-independent persistence of parasitaemia, and suitable exposure patterns qualify dogs as important amplifying reservoirs in rural communities of central and northern Argentina. Such domestic reservoirs are a risk factor for humans living in the same dwelling. Dogs may also serve as natural sentinels in the surveillance phase by helping in detecting the introduction of *T. cruzi* into the domestic cycle (*69, 70*).

Other important domestic reservoirs of the parasite are rabbits and guinea-pigs, as can be seen in various Andean countries. Guinea-pigs, frequently with high rates of *T. cruzi* infection in Bolivia and Peru, play an important epidemiological role as intradomestic reservoirs. They are often reared inside the dwelling, in close contact with humans, and serve as a source of protein. They are sometimes transported alive to distant nonendemic areas, thus contributing to the spread of the parasite.

Marsupials and rodents have also been considered as important synanthropic reservoirs of *T. cruzi*. Less important domestic reservoirs include goats, sheep, and alpacas. Exceptionally, high rates of *T. cruzi* infection have been reported in young swine in rural areas of Pará, Brazil, in association with human cases of Chagas disease and domestic populations of *Panstrongylus geniculatus*.

5.2 Wild reservoirs

More than 180 species or subspecies of small, wild, terrestrial or arboreal mammals belonging to seven orders and 25 families have been found to be naturally infected with *T. cruzi* throughout most of the American continent (see Annex 3). Because of their broad distribution and their rates of *T. cruzi* infection, important infected species or subspecies include: Marsupialia (*Didelphis* spp.), Edentata (*Dasypus novencinctus*), Chiroptera (*Carollia perspicilata*, *Desmodus rotundus*, *Glossophaga soricina*, *Phyllostomus hastatus*), Carnivora (*Dusicyon griseus*, *Eira barbara*, *Nasua* spp.), Rodentia (*Akodon* spp., *Coendu* spp., *Dasyprocta* spp., *Sciurus* spp.), and Primates (*Alouatta* spp., *Ateles* spp., *Cebus* spp., *Saimiri* spp.). Wild reservoirs of epidemiological importance include some edentates, marsupials, and rodents that, because of their habits and favourable local conditions (deforestation, weeding, ploughing), play a significant part in linking the sylvatic and domestic cycles of the parasite.

Three species and subspecies deserve special attention: a marsupial, the opossum (*Didelphis* spp.), an edentate, the armadillo (*Dasypus* spp.), and a rodent, the agouti (*Dasyprocta* spp.). Opossums are probably the most important wild reservoirs because they are omnivorous and very prolific, are highly adaptable ecologically, and have high *T. cruzi* infection rates, with no evidence of disease. They have been found in trees, bromeliads, attics, and roofs. They show long-lasting parasitaemia and can eliminate *T. cruzi* in the urine (*71*). They live in close contact with various triatomine species and are therefore always infected. *T. cruzi* can be detected in the anal glands of naturally infected opossums and this, together with the urinary excretion of the parasite, should favour the oral transmission of *T. cruzi*, as demonstrated both clinically and experimentally, to susceptible mammals, including humans, without the participation of vectors. This mechanism of transmission may account for the outbreaks of Chagas disease in nonendemic areas, as in some places in Brazil. In some parts of the American continent, opossums are highly appreciated as food, and this may sometimes provide another means of oral transmission of *T. cruzi* infection to humans. Alternatively, the infection may be acquired through contact between epidermal erosions or small cuts with blood or other parts of the animals' bodies when they are skinned and prepared for cooking.

Armadillos, which are widely distributed throughout the American continent from the USA to Argentina, are often found infected at rates varying from 5.4 to 55.3%. They are important not only because of their presence near human dwellings, but also because of the special habitat conditions that they offer in their nests to triatomines. Agoutis, distributed from Costa Rica to Ecuador and Brazil, have been found with infection rates ranging from 5.4 to 22.2%.

5.3 Importance of birds and other terrestrial vertebrates

Birds, reptiles, and amphibians are refractory to *T. cruzi* infection because the blood of these animals has a complement-mediated lytic effect on the parasite. They play an important role, however, as feeding sources of many triatomines, particularly in the case of birds. In places where triatomines feed mainly on chickens or pigeons, rates of *T. cruzi* infection are one-fifth of those found in the insects that feed on humans and domestic mammals. It is not clear whether the presence of birds in dwellings is beneficial because of the reduction in the global rate of *T. cruzi* infection in the vectors and because birds eat the bugs, or harmful because a higher total population of insects that have an abundant source of food is maintained.

Many sylvatic birds shelter triatomines in their nests and help to disperse them. Some lizards and toads have been described as feeding sources of certain species of triatomines, such as *T. rubrovaria*, in southern Brazil and Uruguay.

6. Epidemiology and incidence trends

6.1 Modes of transmission and ecological factors

6.1.1 *Transmission by vectors*

T. cruzi is transmitted vectorially through the infected dejections of triatomine bugs. Most cases of Chagas disease can be attributed to the main domiciliated vector species, namely *Panstrongylus megistus*, *Rhodnius prolixus*, *Triatoma brasiliensis*, *T. dimidiata*, *and T. infestans*. These species are characteristic of open environments of Central and South America, either natural areas (savannas and grasslands, grassland–woodland mosaics, dry forest, and the desert and semidesert Andean valleys) or man-made ecotopes.

Recent studies indicate that at least two main groups of *T. cruzi* populations can be found in nature. The first is closely linked to the sylvatic cycle and apparently results in milder infections and morbidity in humans; it is more prevalent in Central and North America. The second is closely related to the domestic cycle and produces major infections and morbidity in humans. There is some evidence that the distribution of such parasite populations is related to the distribution and other characteristics of the vector species, with important epidemiological consequences in human Chagas disease. Current field observations in endemic areas show that the domestic density of infected vectors is closely related to the number of acute cases, mainly in young age groups in which morbidity and mortality are higher. As a consequence of effective vector control, the number of acute cases has decreased markedly or even been reduced to zero in previously highly endemic areas of Argentina, Brazil, Chile, and Uruguay.

6.1.2 *Transmission by blood transfusion*

The rural-to-urban migratory movements that occurred in Latin America from the 1960s onwards changed the traditional epidemiological pattern of *T. cruzi* transmission. What had been primarily a rural infection became an urban one that could be transmitted by blood transfusion. In the past two decades, the numbers of donors with positive serology have been very high in the endemic countries.

At present, in most countries in Latin America, the provision of systems for the screening of blood donors in blood banks has been made compulsory by law in order to prevent the transmission of *T. cruzi* by blood transfusion. Such transmission is not confined to countries where the disease is endemic. The migration of persons infected by *T. cruzi* poses a public health problem even for countries where vectorial transmission of the parasite does not occur, as in Canada and

USA, where transmission of *T. cruzi* by blood products has been reported.

Transfusion Chagas disease depends on a number of epidemiological factors, namely the level of parasitaemia of the donor, the number and volume of transfusions received, the time between blood collection and transfusion, the immunological state of the recipient, etc. The risk of parasite transmission by a single 500-ml transfusion unit of total blood varies from 12 to 20%. *T. cruzi* can also be transmitted by plasma and red blood cell concentrates. Epidemiological data show that transfusion Chagas disease is more common following transfusions of blood from paid donors and in total blood transfusions. As a general rule, the implementation of effective national blood-bank policies results in a drastic reduction in the risk of transfusion Chagas disease.

6.1.3 *Congenital transmission*

The prevalence of *T. cruzi* infection in women varies widely in the different endemic countries. Congenital Chagas disease is by no means restricted to rural areas, but is also reported with increasing frequency in cities where there is no vectorial transmission but to which large numbers of infected women of childbearing age have migrated from the countryside. Cases of congenital Chagas disease have been reported from Argentina, Bolivia, Brazil, Chile, Colombia, Guatemala, Honduras, Paraguay, Uruguay, and Venezuela. One case was also reported in Sweden, in a child of a Latin American immigrant.

The risk of congenital transmission seems to vary according to different epidemiological factors, such as the strain of the parasite, the parasitaemia of the mother, the existence of lesions in the placenta, and the geographical region. This risk has been estimated to range from 1% or less in Brazil to 7% or more in some regions of Bolivia, Chile, and Paraguay. Congenital transmission depends directly on the prevalence of the infection in fertile women who were usually infected by vectorial transmission. In endemic areas subject to vector control, a progressive decrease in congenital disease can be expected over the medium or long term.

6.1.4 *Transmission by organ transplantation*

Patients who have received organs from donors with chronic Chagas disease have experienced acute episodes of the disease, and the parasite has been isolated from peripheral blood. This has occurred most frequently following kidney transplantation. Heart, bone marrow, and pancreas transplantations from both dead and live donors are also possible causes of the transmission of Chagas disease; reports have come from Argentina, Brazil, Chile, and Venezuela (see also pp. 14–17).

6.1.5 *Accidental transmission*

Accidental transmission of human Chagas disease has been reported in several situations, e.g. in laboratories and hospitals of both endemic and nonendemic countries. More than 70 well-documented cases have been recorded in technicians, doctors, and research workers handling different types of contaminated materials, such as triatomine dejections, parasite cultures, and the infected blood of human and animals (see Annex 1).

6.1.6 *Oral transmission*

The oral transmission of Chagas disease has been documented in various epidemics in Brazil, Colombia, and Mexico, following the ingestion of food contaminated with infected triatomines or their dejections.

6.1.7 *Ecological factors*

The epidemiological pattern of *T. cruzi* infections shows that transmission was originally restricted to specific cycles in tropical forest environments, where triatomines would feed on small mammals in broad areas of South America, without humans intervening in the natural cycle. The same situation persists today in the wild. The presence of *T. cruzi* does not seem to significantly affect either the triatomines or the mammals that have been naturally infected. This would suggest a balance between species as a result of long periods of adaptation.

Human Chagas disease developed when humans came into contact with the natural foci of infection and disturbed the environment, with the result that infected triatomines moved into human dwellings. Thus began a process of adaptation to, and domiciliation in human habitations whereby the vectors had direct access to abundant food and were protected from climatic changes and predators.

Humans might then have become infected by accident or as an addition to the already extensive host range of *T. cruzi* that also includes other primates. Environmental factors, such as climatic conditions, influence the rate of increase of triatomine bug populations. Seasonal patterns of abundance and age structure have been determined for domiciliary populations of triatomines. Temperature, relative humidity, and illumination modify triatomine behaviour in relation, for example, to egg laying, ecdysis, reproductive patterns, and feeding habits. In general, the population increases in summer and declines in winter.

Population size depends on the availability of hosts. Where a fixed number of hosts are available, population growth initially occurs, but when the density of triatomines increases, each insect tends to consume less blood because of the competition effect. Finally, the reduction in nutrition results in a decrease in nymphal development and egg laying by female insects, causing the males to fly away. These factors tend to reduce the population density of triatomines.

Triatomines have four mechanisms of dispersion, namely passive and active, and terrestrial and aerial in the case of winged adults. Passive dispersion depends on human behaviour, e.g. passive transport on clothes, vehicles, etc., or the collection of wood in the peridomestic environment. Birds that have triatomine eggs or nymphs in their feathers may also assist dispersion.

Active dispersion by flight is associated with the need for feeding. In domiciliated triatomines, a high population density results in a shortage of food and causes the active dispersion of adults to other houses.

In sylvatic populations, the destruction of the habitat and the disappearance of the hosts can cause the dispersion of triatomines to rural dwellings. The flight distance does not exceed 200 metres for *T. infestans*, but other domestic species such as *R. prolixus*, or sylvatic species such as *T. sordida* and *T. guasayana* are able to fly distances of more than 500 metres.

6.1.8 *Anthropogenic environmental changes*

The adaptation of triatomines to the domestic environment has taken place mainly in the natural open areas of Latin America. Human settlements and colonization have dramatically changed the natural environment, especially through extensive deforestation. The response of triatomine populations to the shortage of blood sources and natural shelter was to colonize human dwellings. On the other hand, in several traditional chagasic areas, agricultural development and other forms of environmental management have led to a considerable simplification of the habitat. This has greatly reduced the risk of invasion of houses and, as a consequence, natural foci of triatomines have ceased to exist. However, where human activities extend into regions such as the Amazon basin, in which many sylvatic species are present, vectorial transmission of *T. cruzi* infection will spread into areas from which it was previously absent.

6.2 Prevalence and geographical distribution of the disease

Data on the prevalence and distribution of Chagas disease improved in quality as a result of the epidemiological studies carried out in the period 1980–1985 in countries where accurate information was not previously available. These studies have provided the only database with which the currently observed reduction in the incidence of human infections can be compared. This reduction in the number of new cases of infection is the consequence of the successful vector-control activities that have led to the interruption of the transmission of Chagas disease in most of Brazil and in Chile and Uruguay.

From countrywide surveys, it was estimated in 1985 that some 100 million people, i.e. 25% of all the inhabitants of Latin America, were at risk of contracting the disease, and the overall prevalence of human *T. cruzi* infection in the endemic countries reached a total of 17.4 million cases. On the basis of studies conducted in Brazil, it is generally accepted that between 10 and 40% of the infected population will develop clinically overt disease; hence it can be assumed that some 4.8–5.4 million people had clinical changes attributable to Chagas disease (see Table 3).

It should be noted that the prevalence and incidence of the disease, as well as the mortality, are constantly changing as a consequence of migration, the effect of control programmes, and changes in socio-economic conditions. Data on the decrease in the incidence of cases of *T. cruzi* infection in the past 10 years as a result of vector control are presented in sections 8.1.6 and 8.1.7.

A brief account of the epidemiological situation in each endemic country is given below.

Argentina. The area of transmission includes the zones north of latitude 44°45′S, covering 60% of the country. The main vector is *T. infestans.* In 1991, the prevalence of infection in 18-year-old males entering military service was 5.8%, while in 1993 it was 1%, i.e. a reduction of 83% in the incidence of infection in this age group. In 1990, there were an estimated 2.33 million infected individuals, of whom 30% developed cardiac clinical manifestations. In 1999, 82% of the endemic area had been treated and was under entomological surveillance; *T. infestans* was found only in 1.2% of houses. In the remaining 18% of the endemic area that was in the attack phase, *T. infestans* was present in 13.5% of houses and in 11.4% of the peridomiciliary area. In 1999, the prevalence of seropositivity in blood banks was 4.1%, compared with 8.7% in 1983. In 13 endemic provinces, 6.5% of 66 800 pregnant women were found to be infected by the parasite.

Table 3
Prevalence of human *T. cruzi* infection in Latin America, 1980–1985

Country	Sample size	Percentage infected	Population at risk (×1000)	Percentage of total population	No. of infected persons (×1000)
Group I[a]					
Argentina	ND	10.0	ND	23	2640
Brazil	1352917[b]	4.2	41054	32	6180
Chile	13514[b]	16.9	11600	63	1460
Honduras	3802	15.2	1824	47	300
Nicaragua	ND	ND	ND	ND	—
Paraguay	4037[b]	21.4	1475	31	397
Uruguay	5924[b]	3.4	975	33	37
Venezuela	5696[b]	3.0	12500	72	1200
Group II[c]					
Bolivia	56000[b]	24.0	1800	32	1300
Colombia	20000	30.0	3000	11	900
Guatemala	3952	16.6	4022	54	1100
Group III[d]					
Costa Rica	1420	11.7	1112	45	130
Ecuador	532	10.7	3823	41	30
El Salvador	524	20.0	2146	45	900
Mexico	ND	ND	ND	ND	—
Panama	1770	17.7	898	47	200
Peru	92	9.8	6766	39	621
Total			*92895*	*25*	*17395*

ND = no data.
[a] Group I: countries in which control programmes are operative and control activities are routine.
[b] Demographic samples statistically representative of country.
[c] Group II: countries in which control programmes have been recently organized and control activities have started.
[d] Group III: countries without control programmes.

Belize. The only vector species of epidemiological importance is *T. dimidiata*, which is restricted to the wild environment. There are sporadic reports of adult insects attracted by light on the periphery of cities and villages. All blood banks are screened and the prevalence among blood donors is less than 1.0%.

Bolivia. T. infestans is the main vector. The endemic area covers 80% of the more than 1 million km^2 of the country, including seven of the nine departments. In 1982, it was estimated that 1.3 million people were infected, and electrocardiographic alterations were found in 26% of them. The triatomine house infestation rate was 41.2% and 30.1% of vectors were infected with *T. cruzi*. More than 50% of blood donors in Santa Cruz were seropositive.

Brazil. The main vector is *T. infestans*, but *T. brasiliensis* and *P. megistus* are also involved in disease transmission. House infestation by *T. infestans* has been reduced: 166 000 insects were captured in the endemic areas by workers in the control programme in 1975, but only 611 were captured in the same areas in 1999, a reduction of 99.7% in the infestation of dwellings by this vector.

In 1975, the endemic area covered 3.6 million km^2, or 36% of the total surface of the country. This is the largest endemic area of the continent, and includes 2493 municipalities of the states of Alagoas, Bahia, Ceará, Espírito Santo, Goiás, Maranhão, Mato Grosso do Sul, Minas Gerais, Pará, Paraíba, Paraná, Pernambuco, Piauí, Rio de Janeiro, Rio Grande do Norte, Rio Grande do Sul, São Paulo, Sergipe, Tocantins, and the Federal District. The percentage of infected individuals who develop a pathological condition varies, but abnormal electrocardiograms are found in 15–30% of seropositive individuals 15–20 years after the initial infection. Most of the digestive cases with megaviscera have been reported from Bahia, Goiás, Minas Gerais, and São Paulo, and make up 10% of the infected population. Infection rates in the age group 0–7 years old have fallen from 5.0% in 1980 to 0.28% in 1999, a reduction of 95% in the incidence of infection in this age group during this period. Furthermore, the prevalence rate of infected blood in blood banks has decreased by 90%, from 7.0% in 1980 to 0.73% in 1998.

Chile. The vector involved in transmission was *T. infestans*, but its numbers have been markedly reduced and vectorial transmission has been interrupted. Transmission occurred in rural and suburban areas of the northern half of the country, between latitudes 18°30′S and 34°36′S. The endemic area covered 350 000 km^2 or 46% of the country. Screening in blood banks has been mandatory in the endemic areas since 1976. Prevalence in blood banks has been reduced to 0.5–2.6% in these areas. An International Commission declared Chile free of transmission of Chagas disease in 1999.

Colombia. The main vector species is *R. prolixus* but *T. dimidiata* is also involved in the transmission of *T. cruzi* to humans. It has been estimated that about 5% of the population is infected and almost 20% are at risk of becoming infected. The departments with the highest endemicity are Arauca, Boyacá, Casanare, Cundinamarca, Meta, Norte de Santander, and Santander. Blood-bank screening was made compulsory in the whole country in 1995 and all donated blood is now screened. Current data show that the prevalence of infected donors is 2.1%. The national vector-control programme was established in 1997.

Costa Rica. The main vector is *T. dimidiata.* The vectors are found in the central plain, extending mainly to the north-west and south-west regions of the country. A seroprevalence of 1–3% was found in some blood banks in the country, which participated in a study in 1987.

Ecuador. The main vector is *T. dimidiata.* Transmission is highest in the coastal region, including the provinces of El Oro, Guayas, and Manabí. Most of the human cases have been diagnosed in Guayaquil, the capital of the province of Guayas. It is estimated that more than 30 000 persons are infected and that 3.8 million people are at risk of contracting the infection. It is also estimated that not more than 1% of blood donors are infected in the country as a whole.

El Salvador. T. dimidiata is the main vector. *R. prolixus* was detected in the country in the 1980s but has disappeared from El Salvador during the past 10 years. Vectors are present in 30–80% of dwellings in rural areas and in small or medium-sized townships. In 1998, the prevalence of the infection in the total population was estimated to be 7.0%.

Guatemala. T. dimidiata is found in 18 of the 22 departments and *R. prolixus* in 5 of them. The infestation rate varies from 12 to 35%. There is a poor blood-bank screening system and the prevalence of seropositive blood donations is up to 8% in some areas.

Honduras. The main vector, *R. prolixus*, is present in 12 departments and the second vector, *T. dimidiata*, in 16. Vectors are present in the departments of Atlantida, Choluteca, Colón, Comayagua, Copán, Cortes, Francisco Morazán, Intibuca, Lempira, Ocotepeque, Olancho, El Paraíso, La Paz, Santa Barbara, Valle, and Yoro. In 1983, the highest infection rates were found in the western and eastern departments and in the southern region. About half the population is estimated to be at risk. Infection rates of 32% or more in the vectors have been reported. The most frequent clinical manifestation is cardiopathy. All blood intended for use in transfusion is tested for infection, and the seroprevalence in blood donors in 1999 was 1.65%, compared with 11% in 1985.

Mexico. Vectors and infected mammals are found in the states of Chiapas, Guanajuato, Guerrero, Hidalgo, Jalisco, México, Michoacán, Morelos, Nayarit, Oaxaca, Puebla, Sonora, Yucatán, and Zacatecas. The prevalence of the disease is highest in the Pacific coast states from Chiapas to Nayarit, in the Yucatán peninsula, and in some central areas of the country. Although most of the human infections and clinical forms in Mexico are considered to be mild, there have been recent reports of some cases of megaviscera. Mexico has not introduced routine screening for *T. cruzi* in blood banks, to which 850 000 donations are made every year and where around 12 760 units of blood could be infected.

Nicaragua. T. dimidiata is present in 14 of the 17 departments and *R. prolixus* in five departments. Blood intended for use in transfusion is tested for infection in 70% of blood banks.

Panama. The main vector is *R. pallescens*, which is found in dwellings in the Chorrera district. This vector is present also in palms in the wild environment. *T. dimidiata* is also an important vector. Screening for infection in blood banks is not compulsory and there are no vector-control programmes.

Paraguay. The main vector is *T. infestans.* Chagas disease is considered to be endemic in all rural areas. Isolated studies suggest that the prevalence of human infections varies from 10% in the Misiones region to 20% in Cordillera Department. The estimated rate of congenital transmission in the country as a whole is 7%. All blood intended for use in transfusion is screened and the seroprevalence in blood donors in 1999 was 5.0%.

Peru. The highest prevalence of human infection is found in the departments of Arequipa, Ica, Moquegua, and Tacna. The southern region, where these departments are located, accounts for 7.7% of the population of the country, with about 394 000 dwellings infested by *T. infestans* and 24 000 infected people. In recent years, several cases of acute Chagas disease have been detected in these departments. Routine screening for *T. cruzi* in blood banks is not carried out. A survey of donors in Lima indicated a prevalence of 2.4% in 1993.

United States of America. Sylvatic vectors and reservoirs of *T. cruzi* have been detected in most of the southern and central states. Although only three autochthonous human infections have been reported, the large number of immigrants from countries to the south, many of whom may be infected with *T. cruzi*, may make it necessary to screen donors for blood transfusion and organ transplantation. *T. barberi, T. lectalana, T. protracta, T. recurva*, and *T. rubides* are the major triatomines, which are usually found in small marsupials captured in wild ecotopes in the southern states, and which eventually became infected by *T. cruzi*.

Uruguay. T. infestans was the only domestic vector. This species was eliminated from houses in the country in 1997. In 1975, the endemic area covered approximately 125 000 km^2 of the country's total area of 187 000 km^2, including the departments of Artigas, Cerro Largo,

Colonia, Durazno, Flores, Florida, Paysandú, Río Negro, Rivera, Salto, San José, Soriano, and Tacuarembó. The prevalence of house infestation rates in the country decreased from 5.65% in 1983 to 0.30% in 1997. The prevalence rate of *T. cruzi* infection decreased in the population as a whole from 5% in 1980 to 0.06% in 1999. Serological surveys carried out in 1997 among young children in the age group 0–4 years showed that Chagas disease transmission had been interrupted.

Venezuela. R. prolixus is the most important vector. The endemic area includes 591 municipalities, covering 700000 km² with an estimated population of 12 million in 1987. The geographical distribution of Chagas disease in Venezuela is restricted to the Andean and coastal regions and, with the exception of the states of Barinas, Lara, and Portuguesa with infestation rates of 2.9%, infestation rates are less than 1.1%. An estimated 71.1% of the endemic areas have been covered by the national control programme and, to date, more than 500000 rural houses have been built, which provide housing for almost 3 million inhabitants. In 1999, the incidence of infected cases in the age group 0–4 years old fell to 0.1% from 1% in 1991. Screening of blood donors has been compulsory since 1988, and current data show very low seroprevalence rates (0.78%).

6.3 Epidemiological trends and changes in the period 1983–2000

By 2000, vector-control activities by countries of the Southern Cone Initiative (Argentina, Bolivia, Brazil, Chile, Paraguay, and Uruguay — see section 8.1) had reduced the incidence of infection in children and young adults by 60% in Paraguay and by 99% in Uruguay, as confirmed by serological data (see Fig. 3 and Table 4). In Venezuela,

Table 4
Human infection by *T. cruzi* and reduction in the incidence of Chagas disease in the countries of the Southern Cone Initiative, 1983–2000

Country	Age group (years)	Infection in 1983 (rates × 100)	Infection in 2000 (rates × 100)	Reduction in incidence (%)	References
Argentina	18	5.8	1.2[a]	80.0	*74, 75*
Brazil	0–4	5.0	0.28	95.0	*76, 77*
Chile	0–10	5.4	0.38	94.0	*78, 79*
Paraguay	18	9.3	3.9	60.0	*75, 80*
Uruguay	6–12	2.5	0.06	99.0	*81, 82*

[a] Data for 1993.

Figure 3
Trends in the reduction of the incidence of infection by _T. cruzi_ in different age groups, Southern Cone Initiative, 1980–2000

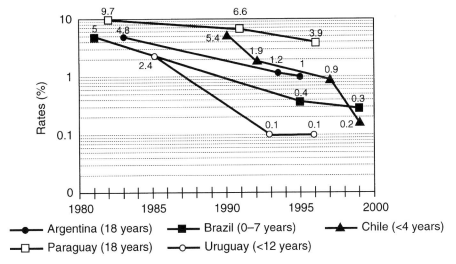

—●— Argentina (18 years)   —■— Brazil (0–7 years)   —▲— Chile (<4 years)
—□— Paraguay (18 years)   —○— Uruguay (<12 years)

WHO 01.20

data on the different age groups show that successive cohorts have had a lower incidence of infection over the period 1959–1999; incidence in the age group 0–9 years fell to 0.1% in 1999.

As previously mentioned, Uruguay was declared free of transmission in 1997 (see p. 67) and Chile in 1999 (see p. 65). Eight out of 12 endemic states of Brazil were certified free of transmission in 2000. The average reduction in incidence in the countries of the Southern Cone Initiative is 94%, so that transmission of Chagas disease in the six countries concerned will be interrupted by 2005 (*72, 73*). The reduction in transmission in these countries has reduced the incidence of Chagas disease in the whole of Latin America by over 65%: from an estimated 700 000 new cases per year in 1983, the incidence has fallen to fewer than 200 000 cases per year in 2000.

Sustained progress has been made since the launching of the Initiative in 1992, as shown by the epidemiological and entomological data.

7. Prevention and control

Chagas disease cannot be eradicated because it is a zoonosis. The large number of animal reservoirs also makes it impossible to eliminate all sources of infection. No drugs are available for large-scale use in reducing, even partially, the chances of transmission and there is no vaccine to protect susceptible individuals. Consequently, the control of vectorial transmission by using insecticides to kill the domiciliated triatomines, and improving houses to make them more difficult for vectors to colonize are the only feasible ways to reduce the opportunities of interaction between humans and vectors.

7.1 Chemical control

Vector control by means of insecticides is effective and has been shown to interrupt transmission because the more anthropophilic species and those that are better adapted to human dwellings or more epidemiologically important, are frequently introduced through passive transportation by humans and are not present outside houses. Species of low vectorial potential and poorly adapted to human dwellings are unlikely to be introduced in areas where they are not native.

It is clear that the use of one particular control method does not exclude the use of others. Chemical control complements house improvement and vice versa.

In the past, there was some resistance to the large-scale use of chemical control measures because of the risk of environmental pollution. In addition, the use of chemicals was believed to provide only temporary control, as opposed to physical control measures such as the improvement of housing. The insecticides currently used (synthetic pyrethroids) have low direct human toxicity, while indirect intoxication by ingestion or contact with the skin is negligible, since the insecticide is applied to surfaces with which human contact is minimal. It has been shown that it is possible to eliminate the main triatomine vectors. The use of residual insecticides is no longer questioned when the domiciliated vector is known to be present and transmission is occurring and must be promptly controlled. Chemical control of the vector is then imperative in view of the severity of the disease. The physical improvement of housing, including the peridomiciliary area, is an alternative when the infestation is geographically limited and residual infestation is persistent.

Chemical control is facilitated if the vector:

— takes a long time to repopulate treated areas;
— lacks mobility and spreads slowly;
— goes through all its development stages in the same habitat and all of them lack resistance to the chemicals used;
— has a low genetic repertoire, and a low ability to develop resistance.

7.1.1 *Introduced and native species*

Different approaches are required to control native species and species introduced into a given area, since the level of control to be achieved is different in each case. With introduced species, the objective can be complete elimination, i.e. the definitive interruption of transmission. With native species, the goal should be to keep housing free from intradomiciliary colonies. The interruption of transmission then requires regular and periodical chemical control and continuous entomological surveillance.

The minimum requirements for domiciliary transmission are: presence of the vector in the house; presence of an infected vector; and colonization of the house by the infected vector. Consequently, if any one of the three conditions is not satisfied, this will be sufficient for control to be achieved.

With introduced species, for which the goal is total elimination, the discovery of a single bug, regardless of its stage of development and whether it is infected, i.e. intra- or peridomiciliary infestation, should be sufficient reason for control to start. With native species, for which the only possible goal of control is to keep houses free of vector colonies, control should be started if intradomiciliary colonization is detected. If nymphs are found inside the house, that alone should be sufficient to prompt immediate control measures. In addition, the operational methodology should vary according to the goals of control.

The same intradomiciliary chemical treatment can be used in areas not previously subject to control, namely the spraying of residual insecticides, in both intradomiciliary and peridomiciliary areas, in two successive selective cycles per infested locality at 6-monthly or yearly intervals. The two requirements that must be satisfied in any such operation are spatial contiguity and temporal continuity.

Before treatment is carried out, entomological research is necessary to obtain information on the number of species present, as well as their dispersion and infestation rates. At the same time, a geographical survey should be undertaken, including a census and identification of local services and resources that may be useful in the operation and in the subsequent entomological surveillance for permanent monitoring of the situation. To that end, the participation of the population and the support of the local health services, as well as other local services and resources, are essential if surveillance is to be effective.

After the initial treatment with two spraying cycles, all subsequent activities will depend on the type of vector prevalent in the area and whether it is an introduced or a native species.

Introduced species
In the Southern Cone Initiative aimed at eliminating *T. infestans* (see section 8.1), elimination was defined as the failure to detect any *T. infestans* for a minimum of 3 years after entomological surveillance had been instituted.

Surveillance must be undertaken after the two initial attack cycles with insecticide, and should preferably combine active search by programme staff and reporting by the local population and health services. If any triatomine is found, even in a single house, the whole locality should undergo a complete course of chemical treatment. Each case should be dealt with in accordance with its particular characteristics. For example, in a very extensive and spatially dispersed locality with only one area vulnerable to triatomine infestation, because of the nature of the houses, only the vulnerable houses would be treated.

The treatment will depend on the epidemiological importance of the species concerned. Thus *T. infestans* is important in the southern cone, while *R. prolixus* is significant in Central America and large parts of the Andean countries where the vectors are strictly domiciliated.

Native species
Native species vary widely in their importance as direct vehicles of Chagas disease infection in the home environment; their control, after the initial attack, therefore requires different strategies. For example, some species may be more or less anthropophilic or adapted to human dwellings, they may have greater or lesser capacity to invade human dwellings, and are infected by the parasite to different degrees.

Various classifications of native species have been proposed on the basis of the interspecies differences. From the point of view of the vector's capacity to establish intradomiciliary colonies, there are at least four possibilities to be considered, depending on the species concerned, as follows:

• Group 1: native species that frequently colonize dwellings, with high or moderate infection rates, e.g. *T. brasiliensis* and *T. dimidiata*.

- Group 2: native species that only infrequently colonize dwellings, with low infection rates and/or little anthropophilism, e.g. *T. maculata* and *T. sordida*.
- Group 3: wild native species with a tendency to become adapted to human dwellings, e.g. *T. rubrovaria*.
- Group 4: strictly wild native species such as *Psammolestes arturi* (see p. 40).

Based on this grouping, the surveillance and treatment provided after the first attack should be as follows:

- Group 1: entomological surveys should be carried out every 2 years, with selective chemical treatment of localities when intradomiciliary colonies of the vector are found.
- Group 2: entomological surveys should also be carried out every 2 years, with selective chemical treatment of homes where intradomiciliary colonies are found. For both groups 1 and 2, massive peridomiciliary infestations indicate the need for the selective spraying of all the houses concerned, even when no colonies are found in a particular house, because of the need to reduce the invasion pressure and prevent the colonization of the house, which may occur when food sources in the peridomicilium are depleted.
- Group 3: surveys may be more widely spaced or surveillance may be carried out only when requested by the population. Treatment can be restricted to houses with proven triatomine colonies.
- Group 4: this does not require any action.

7.1.2 *Inputs and equipment*

Synthetic pyrethroids are the insecticides of choice because of their low toxicity to humans, their powerful triatomicidal effect, and their repellent action. The fact that synthetic pyrethroids act both as strong repellents and insecticides offers the advantage that, even when triatomines are deeply entrenched in walls, they are forced out and then come in contact with the products immediately after their application, when their insecticidal action is strongest. The result is an immediate high mortality rate, so that triatomine colonies are quickly destroyed. Since many products with a similar action are available, it is important to ensure that the minimum effective dose is used. Manually operated, variable-pressure sprayers are most commonly used.

7.1.3 *Programme organization*

Vector control has always taken the form of national campaigns, markedly vertical in character, with the technical decisions being made at the central level and the operations executed only by specialized programme staff. This organizational model ensured that the operations were properly coordinated and that the same methods were used by all. In the case of Chagas disease which, because of its chronicity, produces a very low social demand for medical care services, the impact of the campaigns on vectorial transmission was undeniable.

However, there has been a gradual change in the organizational model, with administrative devolution and operational decentralization coinciding with the need to carry out surveillance activities. This is particularly opportune, since the local level should be responsible for carrying out such activities. On the other hand, there are risks associated with decentralization, such as a loss of visibility and priority because of the need to meet other more immediate or emerging demands. This may lead to a lack of coordination between areas that may have different administrative systems at the municipal, provincial, and state levels.

7.2 Physical control

Physical control means ensuring that houses do not provide favourable conditions for vector colonization either outside or inside. Outside the house, animal shelters must be moved away, and other structures, such as mud ovens, must be improved, e.g. by plastering. Such structures should be the first to be improved since they contain most of the vectors and are the most difficult to spray effectively because of their greater exposure to wind, sun, and rain. The selection of construction materials to be used will depend on their availability and the skills of the community members responsible for house improvement.

Labour requirements should also be taken into account when new construction materials are to be used because skilled labour will then be needed. This not only increases costs, but also takes longer and thus delays the improvement.

Training courses for those interested in improving their living conditions will be necessary. For this purpose, a builder should be employed in every community to teach people the skills required for house improvement. To reduce costs, the use of local materials is strongly recommended.

Entomological surveillance is very important where native species are involved, and communities must maintain continuous surveillance to ensure the early detection of reinfestation.

Housing improvement not only improves people's health and quality of life but also protects against Chagas disease. Improvements such as replacing the flooring or roofing and plastering the walls are effective in controlling vector species such as *T. dimidiata* and *R. prolixus.* The management of the peridomiciliary area reduces the chances of colonization by species that prefer outdoor ecotopes where they are associated with domestic animals. Some houses may have to be replaced if they have been identified as foci that maintain residual triatomine colonies in certain localities because of their construction or location.

As a rule, housing improvement is indicated in areas where native species with proven vectorial capability are present in high densities in the wild. It is obviously desirable when economically feasible, but should not be allowed to delay chemical control of the vectors.

The structure of rural houses makes them particularly vulnerable to infestation with triatomine bugs. Mud walls, poor plaster, cracks, crevices, and thatched roofs offer many hiding places. In rural areas, in addition, there is a close association between humans and domestic animals, and the latter provide a large and readily available source of blood. This continued access to food allows triatomines to reach high densities. Interruption of vectorial transmission is achieved mainly by means of insecticide spraying campaigns and cleaning the insides of dwellings.

Housing improvement with local labour and construction materials has been used in a project in Venezuela as an alternative method of interrupting transmission since the late 1950s. Experience in that country has demonstrated the importance of community participation in housing improvement for low-income families; an educational manual is used in conjunction with methods of meeting local costs, including a system of credits for the purchase of local materials. No evidence of bug infestation was found in the communities concerned after the project was completed. A multidisciplinary pilot project with community-based vector-control strategies that combined housing improvement with insecticide application has also been carried out in Bolivia. In this project, housing improvement, insecticide spraying, and health education were combined. In Honduras, insecticide application was followed by housing improvement and education.

In Paraguay, a multidisciplinary project that took account of the sociocultural values of the traditional house style was carried out in three endemic communities. The impact on vector control and on *T. cruzi* transmission was measured using changes in house infestation rates and in human seropositivity rates for *T. cruzi* infection. This project showed that insecticide application in domestic and peridomestic areas was crucial in keeping houses free of triatomines.

For native vector species, the goal is to keep housing free from intradomiciliary colonies. This depends not only on spraying insecticides or on house improvement but also on the surveillance of residual and persistent bug infestation. Community education on the role played by the vectors in disease transmission is essential in ensuring that people understand the importance of keeping houses in good condition and are on the alert for triatomine infestations, which must be reported to the health authorities so that the reinfested houses can be sprayed.

7.3 Health education and community participation

In addition to house improvement, other measures are needed to keep villages free of triatomines, including a dynamic and permanent education programme to provide information about the disease, the necessary control measures, and the importance of house maintenance in avoiding reinfestation. Families must accept that housing improvement is necessary and should be involved in decisions about the areas to be improved as well as the construction materials to be used. The educational process that precedes housing improvement is long but essential. Having learned that the presence of triatomines represents a health risk for their community, families that commit themselves to carrying out housing improvement must also persuade other families to do the same.

Communication and education have always had and will continue to have a special role in the control and surveillance of triatomine vectors. In Uruguay, where successful control has resulted in the elimination of *T. infestans*, communication and education have been crucial in maintaining the interest of the population. The radio, which is widely listened to in rural areas, and education through local schools were considered to be the most effective means of communication. Communication via community leaders was also considered important.

7.4 Improvement of living conditions

The cleaning of the inside and outside of houses as well as of places where animals are kept must be encouraged. The advantages of good living habits should be discussed at community meetings. Frequent cleaning of the house, and particularly of bedrooms, the kitchen, and structures outside the house, is necessary, together with constant active searches for bugs in places where they are likely to reappear. If reinfestation occurs, the householder must report it to the designated surveillance post so that control measures can be taken. Supervision visits to such posts by programme staff, as well as frequent educational meetings with the community, are also needed.

7.5 Programme implementation in the context of primary health care

Since the main epidemiological features of Chagas disease and the tools available for control and treatment are well known, there is general agreement on the appropriate measures to be carried out through an integrated approach, involving the control of both vectors and blood banks together with medical and social assistance to infected individuals. Local physicians and institutions have a major role to play in the early detection and control of the disease.

According to the results of pilot projects in Argentina, Bolivia, and Brazil, the carrying out of integrated control activities under the primary health care strategy depends on there being a health services structure, local commitment, and close supervision in the area concerned. In addition, experience shows that, for vector-control activities, vertical programmes are highly effective and easy to carry out. However, in the surveillance phase, with low triatomine densities, vertical programmes have low sensitivity and are too expensive, and thus impossible to sustain for any length of time.

In the new context of decentralized operations, what is most important is to ensure that the control of Chagas disease is given the necessary priority. This can be particularly difficult when a level of control has been achieved that is sufficient to interrupt transmission. It is then not feasible, or even reasonable, to think in terms of surveillance that is not integrated into a larger system in which the presence of the Chagas disease vector is only one of the elements to be monitored.

7.6 Evaluation of vector resistance to insecticides

Before 1975, the insecticides and their formulations used for Chagas vector control were evaluated directly in field trials without previous laboratory bioassays performed with triatomines under standard conditions. The unexpected failure of the field use of DDT in the initial campaigns for the control of triatomines demonstrated the importance of such bioassays as a first step in assessing insecticide efficacy. The low triatomicidal efficacy of DDT was later shown by research on nymphs of *T. infestans* in Latin American laboratories to be the consequence of particular degradation pathways and delayed penetration.

In 1975, the first standard protocol for use in the measurement of triatomicidal activity in the laboratory was developed, and made it possible to determine the toxicity of commercial insecticides to *T. infestans*.

7.6.1 *Laboratory bioassays*

The term "laboratory bioassay" covers all tests in which the toxicity of an active substance or its formulation is measured by reference to standardized insect colonies. Evaluation of the toxicological effect of insecticides and their formulations in the laboratory is based on the measurement of the response of an insect strain to such products. The toxic response (the end-point of the intoxication process) is chosen according to the mode of action of the insecticides. The lethal response (death as the end-point) is used in most bioassays. When death is the end-point, the toxicity of the product to an insect species is usually expressed in terms of the lethal dose or concentration that kills 50% of a particular population of the insect species used in the test (LD_{50} or LC_{50}).

It is sometimes necessary to define an end-point other than death. The use of insect growth regulators, and particularly juvenoid compounds, results in the retention of juvenile characters after the ecdysis of nymph V of *T. infestans*. For these compounds, toxicity is expressed in terms of the dose or concentration that affects the morphology of 50% of treated insects. Hyperactivity, suppression of food intake, repellence, loss of coordination, and paralysis have also been used as end-points in measuring the toxicity of different compounds to *T. infestans* (*83*).

In 1994, a standard protocol for insecticide bioassays in triatomines was developed by WHO (*84*), which made it possible for the results of the determination of insecticide activity obtained by different laboratories to be compared. The WHO protocol has been used mainly in the measurement of the LD_{50} values of the most important pyrethroid compounds used in Latin American vector-control programmes. The protocol also specifies the methodology to be used to quantify the insecticidal effect and residual activity of insecticide formulations. Values of LD_{50} and LC_{50} for pyrethroids obtained with the WHO protocol and recommended field concentrations are shown in Table 5.

7.6.2 *Insecticidal effect of formulations*

The formulation process of an insecticide improves its storage, handling, and application properties and its efficacy and safety. The term "formulation" is usually reserved for commercial products before

Table 5
Formulations, LD$_{50}$, LC$_{50}$, and field concentrations of pyrethroids commonly used for indoor spraying against triatomines, 1997

Insecticide	Formulation	LD$_{50}$ (µg/g body weight)	LC$_{50}$ (µg/cm^2 of glass)	Field concentration (mg active ingredient/m^2 treated surface
Deltamethrin	Suspension concentrate	1.54	0.17	25.00
λ-Cyhalothrin	Wettable powder	0.11	0.26	30.00
Cypermethrin	Wettable powder	2.86	—	125.00
β-Cyfluthrin	Suspension concentrate	0.32	0.14	25.00
β-Cypermethrin	Suspension concentrate	1.56	0.21	50.00

actual use and does not include the final dilution in the application equipment. After an active principle has been selected in the light of the results of the laboratory bioassay, the choice of formulation will depend on the toxicological, physical, and chemical properties, the type of application, and the cost. The main technical factors taken into account in the use of the formulation for the control of triatomines are safety, ease of application, and residual effect. The formulation itself should be tested in the laboratory in order to establish its efficacy and residual activity. Until the late 1980s, the most common formulations were wettable powders and emulsifiable concentrates. Flowable formulations have been used recently and are considered to be the best option in national vector-control programmes.

The methodology used in evaluating insecticidal activity is based on the exposure of triatomines to a standardized surface treated with the formulation concerned.

7.6.3 *Resistance and tolerance*

An extensive programme of monitoring resistance to insecticides in Latin America is now possible through the application of the WHO protocol. Laboratory methods of measuring triatomine susceptibility to insecticides are used to monitor the emergence and evolution of insect resistance.

Resistance to dieldrin in *R. prolixus* in Venezuela, reported in 1971, is the first well-documented example of field resistance in triatomines. A strain of *R. prolixus* from Carabobo showed resistance to pyrethroids in ratios ranging from 12.4 for cypermethrin to 4.5 for lambda-cyhalothrin. This was surprising, as *R. prolixus* was controlled in

Venezuela with organochlorines. However, *R. prolixus* might have been exposed to pyrethroids because of their intensive use for mosquito control in Carabobo State (*85*).

Resistance is a preadaptative phenomenon where genes responsible for defence against insecticides are present at very low frequency in wild insect populations. Insecticide use then encourages the predominance of those insect populations with genes able to confer resistance. In contrast, in the case of tolerance, the wild strain of a particular insect species already has some kind of defence mechanism against one or more insecticides. Tolerance to insecticides in the triatomine species needs further study because of its potential relevance to control programmes.

Up to now, there is no evidence that such resistance to, or tolerance of, insecticides has reduced the efficacy of control programmes based on insecticide spraying. However, resistance must be closely monitored in order to optimize the control of triatomines.

8. Subregional initiatives for the interruption of transmission

The World Health Assembly, on 16 May 1998, adopted resolution WHA51.4 in which it expressed its satisfaction with the progress made in the countries of the Southern Cone Initiative (see below) in eliminating the transmission of Chagas disease and acknowledged the decision of the Andean and Central American countries to launch similar initiatives (see sections 8.2 and 8.3, respectively). It also called on the Member States concerned to determine the extent of the disease, including the distribution, behaviour, and sensitivity to insecticides of the various vectors (see also p. 92).

8.1 Southern Cone Initiative

8.1.1 *Situation analysis*

The extensive knowledge available on the control of the mechanisms of transmission of *T. cruzi* — vectorial and through blood transfusions — was for many years not enough to secure the political and financial support needed for the implementation of control programmes. The fact that Chagas disease is a chronic disease with a long period of evolution and almost no clinical symptoms in its acute and indeterminate phases, together with its presence almost exclusively in rural populations with little political leverage explains the lack of interest in its control.

The toxicity to triatomines of hexachlorocyclohexane, also known as benzene hexachloride (BHC), was demonstrated in 1947, and in the field in Argentina and Brazil in 1948. Nevertheless, regular control programmes were implemented in both countries only in the early 1960s. These two countries were therefore pioneers in the large-scale control of vectorial transmission. Initially, however, the activities did not have the required temporal continuity, spatial contiguity, and sustainability, so that the results were both limited and temporary. The main reason for this was the irregular provision of resources, which were insufficient to provide complete coverage of the endemic areas. Regular control activities in the Southern Cone countries were extended to Chile and Uruguay in the 1980s and later to Bolivia and Paraguay.

In 1991, Argentina, Brazil, Chile, and Uruguay were regularly carrying out control activities, while Bolivia and also Peru, which has high levels of infestation by *T. infestans* in its southern departments, did not have properly structured programmes. At that time, infestation rates in Brazil, Chile, and Uruguay were already quite low in most of the areas with endemic *T. infestans*, but there were still areas of high infestation in Argentina, and surveillance was carried out only in part of the endemic area.

8.1.2 *The formal decision*

In July 1991, the Ministers of Health of Argentina, Bolivia, Brazil, Chile, Paraguay, and Uruguay met in Brasilia and decided to implement a strategy aimed at the elimination of Chagas disease by interruption of vectorial transmission and the systematic screening of blood donors. The objectives included the elimination of *T. infestans* from both dwellings and the peridomiciliary environment in endemic areas, and the elimination of transmission of the infection through blood transfusions by improving the screening of blood donors. The success achieved in the state of São Paulo, Brazil, showed that this was feasible; the objectives were achieved within 10 years (*77, 79, 82*).

8.1.3 *Strategies and methods*

In the light of the different epidemiological situations and organizational structures of the control programmes in each country, it was agreed that countries should adopt common concepts, indicators, and operational standards. The definition adopted for the elimination of *T. infestans* was the "lack of detection of any specimen of *T. infestans* in the intradomiciles for a minimum period of three years in an area with entomological surveillance established and operative using the research techniques available". The agreed strategy to eliminate *T. infestans* was chemical treatment with residual in-secticides, in 6-monthly cycles, based on the minimum information required, namely the infestation rates in the localities used as operational units. The two initial attack cycles with insecticide must cover all the infested localities. Because the concept of elimination was based on the finding of the insect, the need for an entomological surveillance system right from the start of the operations was stressed. Community participation in the surveillance activities and the support of the local health services were also deemed crucial to guarantee the sustainability of the activities. The criteria needed for the certification of the elimination of *T. infestans*, as well as the indicators (see Box 2), information system, and methodology to be used for entomological and epidemiological surveillance, were also agreed (*84*). The guidelines described above have been used by all the countries involved and as a model by the Andean and Central American countries.

8.1.4 *Intercountry mechanisms*

Two mechanisms were established for the monitoring and evaluation of vector-control activities, of which the first is the annual meeting of

---

Box 2

Entomological indicators for Chagas disease control

Operational
Dispersion: the numbers of vectors in various localities (dispersion) are used to determine the general areas in which vectors are present and to define those in which control measures are necessary.

$$\frac{\text{Number of infested localities}}{\text{Number of localities investigated}} \times 100$$

Evaluation and follow-up
House infestation: the numbers of vectors in houses (infestation) are used to determine the distribution and density of infestation in a given area. This is the main operational indicator.

$$\frac{\text{Number of infested houses}}{\text{Number of houses investigated}} \times 100$$

Intradomiciliary infestation:

$$\frac{\text{Number of infested intradomiciles}}{\text{Number of intradomiciles investigated}} \times 100$$

Box 2 (*continued*)

Peridomiciliary infestation:

$$\frac{\text{Number of infested peridomiciles}}{\text{Number of peridomiciles investigated}} \times 100$$

Natural infection (by T. cruzi):

$$\frac{\text{Number of infected triatomines}}{\text{Number of triatomines examined}} \times 100$$

Colonization: separate indicators can be calculated for intradomiciliary and peridomiciliary colonization.

$$\frac{\text{Number of houses with triatomine nymphs}}{\text{Number of houses examined}} \times 100$$

Density: separate indicators can be calculated for intradomiciliary and peridomiciliary density.

$$\frac{\text{Number of triatomines captured}}{\text{Number of houses examined}} \times 100$$

Surveillance

These indicators are used in the validation of the surveillance system, in terms of the levels of coverage and programme output and quality.

Coverage:

$$\frac{\text{Number of infested localities under surveillance}}{\text{Number of previously infested localities}} \times 100$$

Output: refers to established notification units.

$$\frac{\text{Number of productive notification units}}{\text{Number of notification units established}} \times 100$$

Quality:

$$\frac{\text{Number of positive localities for traces of triatomines}}{\text{Number of localities with positive notifications}} \times 100$$

$$\frac{\text{Number of positive localities for triatomine detection}}{\text{Number of localities with positive notifications}} \times 100$$

$$\frac{\text{Number of positive localities for a particular species}}{\text{Number of localities with positive notifications}} \times 100$$

$$\frac{\text{Number of treated localities}}{\text{Number of localities with positive notifications}} \times 100$$

$$\frac{\text{Number of houses treated}}{\text{Number of positive houses notified}} \times 100$$

the Intergovernmental Commission consisting of technical representatives of each Ministry of Health; this is held in member countries in rotation. These meetings serve various purposes, including the review of the progress made towards the goals established, and the discussion of issues arising from fieldwork and requiring field research and operational decisions.

The second mechanism, which has given political sustainability to the Initiative and at the same time promoted a permanent exchange of experience at the technical level, consists of the periodic in-situ evaluations made by international evaluation missions of experts from both the endemic and nonendemic countries of the region. These external evaluations review progress and recommend corrective action for the future, if necessary. There is also a bilateral mechanism for reviewing the situation in frontier areas and for dealing with problems common to more than one country.

8.1.5 *Resources*

In order to accomplish the goals set by the Ministers of Health in 1991, it was decided that funds from national sources should be made available. The budgetary commitments made have been honoured, and in the period 1991–1999 more than US$ 350 million have been invested in Chagas disease control by the countries of the Initiative.

8.1.6 *Results*

As previously mentioned, Uruguay was certified free of vectorial and transfusional transmission of Chagas disease in 1997 (*82*), while Chile interrupted transmission in 1999 (*79*) and eight of the 12 endemic states of Brazil were certified free of transmission in 2000 (*77, 86*). Seroepidemiological surveys in young age groups in Uruguay (*87*) and Chile (*88*) have confirmed that transmission has been interrupted in these two countries.

There is evidence that vectorial transmission has been interrupted in the provinces of Jujuy, La Pampa and La Rioja in Argentina. In Bolivia, the national vector-control programme started activities in 1999 and, of the 700 000 houses that it is estimated need to be sprayed, more than 97 000 have been treated with insecticides. In Paraguay, the interruption of transmission should be achieved in 4 years, provided that funds for vector control continue to be available.

Remarkable progress has been made with regard to the transmission of *T. cruzi* through blood transfusion. Specific legislation requiring the serological screening of donors was introduced in all the countries of the Initiative to reduce the transmission of Chagas disease in this way.

The impact of control on the health of the population will be seen in the years to come, but 325 000 new annual cases of infection by *T. cruzi* have already been prevented by the control activities in the contries of the Southern Cone Initiative since 1995, and 127 000 cases of cardiomyopathy and sudden death have also been prevented. From the economic point of view, these countries have saved more than US$ 1140 million in health care expenditure and social security costs.

8.1.7 *Overall impact of the Initiative in the region*

As previously mentioned, the average reduction of the incidence of Chagas disease in the countries of the Southern Cone Initiative is 94%, so that incidence of the disease in the whole of Latin America has been reduced by over 65%. From an estimated 700 000 new cases per year in 1990, incidence has fallen to fewer than 200 000 cases per year in 2000 (see Table 6 and p. 68).

At present, the major challenge is to ensure the sustainability of the programme both in an epidemiological context (where infection with *T. cruzi* has been greatly reduced) and in a political–institutional context of health sector reforms in which the decentralization of activities may mean that the priority accorded to them may be reduced.

Maintaining this priority will depend on social demand. Under the new institutional order, Chagas disease control must be integrated into other services and programmes, becoming part of a broader scheme for meeting the health needs of the population. In these circumstances, the significant progress made so far towards the elimination of Chagas disease must be continued by the integrated activities.

Table 6

Changes in epidemiological parameters due to the interruption of transmission and decrease in incidence, 1990–2000, in the countries of the Southern Cone Initiative

Epidemiological parameter	1990	2000	References
No. of deaths per year	>45 000	21 000	*89, 90*
No. of cases of human infection	16–18 million	18 million	*89*
No. of new cases per year	700 000	200 000	*78, 79, 81*
Distribution	18 countries	15 countries[a]	

[a] Transmission was interrupted in Uruguay in 1997, in Chile in 1999, and in most of Brazil in 2000.

The model implemented in the Southern Cone has already been adapted to the two similar initiatives in the Andean countries and Central America (see sections 8.2 and 8.3, respectively).

8.1.8 *Cost–effectiveness studies in Brazil*

The Brazilian Ministry of Health carried out a cost–effectiveness and cost–benefit analysis of the Chagas disease control programme in Brazil. Because of the chronic nature of the disease and its long duration, a period of 21 years was chosen for the analysis. For the period 1975–1995, data from a number of different sources were analysed (*91*). Effectiveness was defined in terms of various parameters, of which the most important was the measurement of the burden of disease prevented in disability-adjusted life-years (DALYs). From 1975 to 1995, the programme prevented an estimated 89% of potential disease transmission, i.e. 2 339 000 new infections and 337 000 deaths. This represents a prevented loss of 11 486 000 DALYs, 31% from deaths prevented and 69% from disability prevented, showing the major contribution of disability to the overall burden attributable to Chagas disease.

The estimated benefits (expenditures prevented) of the programme were US$ 7500 million, 63% of the savings being on health care expenditures and 37% on social security expenditures (disability insurance and retirement pensions). The cost–effectiveness analysis demonstrated that, for each US$ 39 spent by the programme, 1 DALY was gained. This places the programme and its activities in the category of very highly cost-effective interventions. The results of the cost–benefit analysis also showed savings of US$ 17 for each dollar spent on prevention, demonstrating that the programme is a health investment that gives a good return. A similar analysis of other diseases with socioeconomic causes showed that the decline in Chagas disease infection rates is due to the preventive activities, and not to the general improvement in living conditions and development.

8.2 Andean Initiative

8.2.1 *Andean Pact agreement*

During a meeting of representatives of the Ministers of Health of the Andean Pact countries held in 1997 in Santa Fé de Bogotá, Colombia, within the framework of the Hipolito Unanue Agreement, it was decided to establish an Andean Initiative modelled on the Southern Cone Initiative with the aim of interrupting the vectorial and transfusional transmission of Chagas disease in the subregion. The target date for the interruption of transmission in the subregion is 2010. The situation in the different countries is summarized below.

Colombia. The departments with the highest endemicity are Arauca, Boyacá, Casanare, Cundinamarca, Meta, Norte de Santander, and Santander. It has been estimated that about 5% of the Colombian population is infected and close to 20% are at risk of becoming infected, depending on the geographical distribution of the vectors. *R. prolixus* is the principal and most common vector of *T. cruzi* in Colombia. The national control programme was conceived as an integral programme, with the following components: vector control, the control of blood transfusion, the control of congenital transmission, the treatment of infected patients, and a rural housing improvement programme. Compulsory screening of blood donors for *T. cruzi* began in 1995 and all blood donors are now screened.

The national programme was started in 1997. The first exploratory phase of the programme — to identify the areas of transmission — has been completed, and covered 55% of the total endemic area of Colombia. The results indicated a high risk of transmission in several municipalities in the departments of Arauca, Boyacá, Casanare, Cundinamarca, Norte de Santander and Santander.

Ecuador. The main endemic area covers the provinces of El Oro in the south-western coastal region and Guayas and Manabí in the central and northern Pacific coastal areas. *T. dimidiata* and *R. prolixus* are the most important vectors. It has been estimated that approximately 3.8 million people are at risk of acquiring Chagas disease and more than 30 000 individuals are currently infected. Efforts have been made at the national level to control the transmission of Chagas disease by transfusion and all blood donors are screened.

Peru. *T. infestans* is prevalent in the departments of Arequipa, Ica, Moquegua, and Tacna. It has been estimated that 6.7 million people are at risk of acquiring the infection and 680 000 are infected with *T. cruzi* in the whole country.

Venezuela. The control programme was officially established in 1966 with the objective of interrupting intradomestic transmission through vector control by insecticide spraying. A programme for the improvement of rural housing, begun in the 1960s, assists rural inhabitants to replace palm roofs, plaster adobe walls, and concrete earthen floors. In addition, routine screening for *T. cruzi* in blood banks was begun in 1988.

In children under 10 years of age, the seroprevalence rates for *T. cruzi* infection have declined steadily over the past 40 years from 20.5% (1958–1968) to 3.9% (1969–1979) and then to 1.1% (1980–1989) and to 0.8% at present (1990–1999). The incidence of infection in the age group 0–4 years has been reduced by 90% to less than 1.0% over the period 1990–1999. The geographical distribution of *T. cruzi* transmission is today largely restricted to the states of Barinas, Lara, and Portuguesa (*92*).

8.3 Central American Initiative

8.3.1 *Central American agreement*

Resolution No. 13 of the XIII Meeting for the Health Sector of Central America (RESSCA), held in Belize in 1997, launched the Central American Initiative for the control of vectoral and transfusional transmission of *T. cruzi.* The objectives of the Initiative are the elimination of *R. prolixus* in El Salvador, Guatemala, Honduras, and Nicaragua (since it is an introduced and strictly domiciliary species), the reduction of the infestation and colonization indexes of *T. dimidiata* (an autochthonous species) throughout Central America, and the screening of all blood donors.

An Intergovernmental Commission of the Central American Initiative meets annually to review progress in vector and blood-bank control.

8.3.2 *Situation analysis*

R. prolixus, *T. dimidiata*, and *R. pallescens* are the main vectors in Central America. Of these, *R. prolixus* is the most efficient and responsible for the majority of human infections. It is found in El Salvador, Guatemala, Honduras, and Nicaragua, always strictly associated with human dwellings in rural areas.

T. dimidiata, the autochthonous species in Central America, is considered to be the next most important vector. It can be found in both domiciliary and peridomiciliary areas, as well as in the wild. It also has an urban distribution, which makes it an important vector in many cities of Central America. *T. dimidiata* is the species responsible for transmission in Costa Rica, and is the only important species in Belize. *R. pallescens* is considered the most important species in Panama.

Chagas disease is a major public health problem in Central America, especially in El Salvador, Guatemala, Honduras, and Nicaragua. The estimated prevalence of infection among the population of these four countries is 7.0%. Chronic cardiopathy is the most frequently observed manifestation. In Honduras, 20.0% of chronic cardiopathies are chagasic, and 36.0% of pacemakers implanted in Guatemala and Honduras are for arrhythmias of chagasic etiology (*93*).

Until the 1970s, only isolated efforts were made to control vectorial transmission in the various Central American countries, but these were unsuccessful because of the lack of continuity. Prevalence studies in the general population have been carried out in Guatemala, Honduras, and Panama, and in children less than 12 years old in El Salvador, Guatemala, and Nicaragua. All blood donors are screened in El Salvador and Honduras, but only some are screened in Guatemala and Nicaragua. In Costa Rica and Panama, the percentage of donors screened is less than 10%.

The elimination of *R. prolixus* from Guatemala, Honduras, and Nicaragua by 2005 is feasible. The surveillance of *T. dimidiata*, a sylvatic vector that also colonizes houses, will need to be continued for some time to come.

At present, no routine vector-control activities are being carried out in Belize, Costa Rica, or Panama.

9. Development of human resources

The UNDP/World Bank/WHO Special Programme for Research and Training in Tropical Diseases (TDR) was established to promote and fund research training and institution strengthening designed to increase the participation of developing countries in the development and use of new tools for the prevention and control of tropical diseases. Its long-term mission is to foster self-reliance in the endemic countries by building a critical mass of human resources and scientific knowledge in biomedical and social sciences, in a research environment that is able to respond to public health research needs. Partnerships, networking, and the promotion of equal opportunities in endemic countries constitute the core of the TDR strategy.

Over the years, TDR has shown great flexibility and has used different approaches in meeting a variety of research needs, taking into account the differences in the research capability of the various endemic countries.

During the period 1975–1999, TDR invested US$ 8.7 million in research on Chagas disease, both by individuals and by institutions, representing 27% of its total investment (US$ 32 million) in capacity-building activities in tropical diseases control in Latin America for this period.

This investment has met countries' demands and increased the potential for further research capacity development in Latin America. Argentina and Brazil alone accounted for about 65% of the funding for capacity building for Chagas disease control. Given the existence of an established core of scientists and research institutions concerned with Chagas disease in Latin America, most of the funding was allocated to more advanced laboratory-oriented research development or complex population-based epidemiological investigations, rather than to elementary training. During the same period, additional support was provided through the Chagas Disease Steering Committee and the Task Force on Operational Research for Chagas Disease. All this financial assistance has contributed to improving the quality of research on Chagas disease in Latin America and to developing expertise in the fields of epidemiology, immunology, biochemistry, molecular biology, genomics, and molecular entomology.

10. Research priorities

The Committee considers that the following are the most important research priorities, given the large extent to which Chagas disease is now controlled.

10.1 Clinical pathology and diagnostic tests

10.1.1 Clinical pathology

- Analytical epidemiological case–control studies with standardized protocols should be carried out in different countries to identify factors related to the parasite, the host and the environment that are responsible for the different clinical forms of the disease.
- Prognostic markers should be developed to study the transformation of the indeterminate form of the disease into the cardiac or digestive form.
- Studies should be carried out on the prevalence and incidence of congenital transmission and the parasite strains involved.

10.1.2 Diagnostic tests

- Multicentre studies should be carried out on the sensitivity and specificity of PCR in different countries in which the prevalence of infection differs.
- Multicentre studies should be carried out on the sensitivity and specificity of non-conventional serological tests in different countries in which the prevalence of infection differs.

10.1.3 New tools for use in evaluating vector control

- Sensitive tools should be developed for the detection of vectors where triatomine density is low.

- Studies should be carried out to characterize intradomiciliary and sylvatic populations of triatomines and to assess the efficacy of insecticides.
- The distribution and vectorial capacity of emerging triatomine species and their relationship to parasite strains should be studied.
- The dynamics of the native species should be investigated with the aim of achieving prompt intervention.
- Studies should be undertaken of the vector peridomiciliary ecotope as a link between the sylvatic and peridomiciliary infection cycles.
- Vector resistance and the efficacy of insecticides in national control programmes and the impact of these programmes should be monitored and evaluated.
- The influence of climatic changes on the populations of vectors should be determined.

10.2 Biochemistry, functional genomics, and drug development

- The information generated in the *Trypanosoma cruzi* genome project should be used in the following research areas:

   (i)   the search for new targets for drug development;
   (ii) the identification of structural and functional components involved in the host–parasite interaction;
   (iii) the achievement of a better understanding of the biological properties of the parasite strains;
   (iv) the study of genetic markers for drug resistance in parasite strains.

10.3 Social and economic research

- The social communication techniques involved in community participation during the vector surveillance phases that follow the interruption of the transmission of the disease should be evaluated.

11. Recommendations

1. The progress made in interrupting the transmission of Chagas disease in several countries of Latin America in the past 20 years has been remarkable, and continued support should be provided to the national control programmes and to research institutions in the endemic countries so as to meet the goal of eliminating transmission of the disease by the year 2010, as required by World Health Assembly resolution WHA51.14.

2. The endemic countries should continue their vector-control and surveillance activities irrespective of the extent to which vectorial

transmission has been interrupted. Those countries that have achieved interruption should maintain national vector-surveillance activities for whatever period of time is necessary to ensure that their territory remains free of intradomiciliary vector transmission of the disease.

3. The endemic countries should continue their programmes for the screening of blood banks for *Trypanosoma cruzi* so as to ensure that the transmission of the parasite through blood transfusion is also interrupted.

4. National efforts should be made to ensure that infected individuals in the early indeterminate phase of the disease are treated with the only currently available drug (benznidazole). Individuals living in areas where vectorial transmission has been interrupted should be treated so as to avoid reinfection. At the same time, research aimed at developing new effective drugs should be continued.

5. National systems and methods should be developed and implemented for the quality control of diagnostic reagents and insecticides before their approval for use in clinical management, blood-bank screening, and spraying activities.

6. Epidemiological and clinical studies on congenital Chagas disease should be encouraged in those countries that have achieved the interruption of the vectorial transmission of the disease.

7. The different methods of implementing the available validated vector control and blood-bank control strategies should be subjected to economic analysis by the ministries of health of the endemic countries.

8. Continued support should be given to research and training activities carried out by WHO, including those of the UNDP/World Bank/WHO Special Programme for Research and Training in Tropical Diseases.

Acknowledgements

The Expert Committee acknowledges the valuable contributions of the following persons, who helped to provide a basis for its discussions and report: Dr D. Akhavan, Ministry of Health, Brasilia, Brazil; Dr J. Altclas, Bone Marrow Transplant Unit, Antartida Sanatorium, Buenos Aires, Argentina; Professor Z. Andrade, Gonçalo Muñiz Research Centre–FIOCRUZ, Salvador, Bahia, Brazil; Dr F. Balderrama, Centre for Health in the Home, Cochabamba, Bolivia; Dr R. Carcavallo, Oswaldo Cruz Foundation, Entomology Department, Rio de Janeiro, Brazil; Dr C. Cordon-Rosales, Centre for Health Studies, University of the Valley of Guatemala, Guatemala City, Guatemala; Dr L. Diotaiuti, René Rachou Research Centre–FIOCRUZ, Belo Horizonte, Brazil; Dr R. Docampo, Laboratory of Molecular Parasitology, University of Illinois, Urbana, IL, USA; Dr J. P. Dujardin, Department of Tropical Diseases, Bolivian High-Altitude Biology Institute (IBBA), La Paz, Bolivia; Dr D. Feliciangeli, University of Carabobo, Venezuela; Dr O. Fernandez, Department of Tropical Medicine, Oswaldo Cruz Foundation, Rio de Janeiro,

Brazil; Dr A. Fragata Filho, Dante Pazzanese Institute of Cardiology, São Paulo, Brazil; Dr H. Freilij, "Dr Ricardo Gutierrez" Children's Hospital, Buenos Aires, Argentina; Dr S. M. Gonzalez-Cappa, Faculty of Medicine, University of Buenos Aires, Buenos Aires, Argentina; Dr M. L. Higuchi, University of São Paulo Medical School, São Paulo, Brazil; Dr C. Jaramillo, Centre for Research on Tropical Microbiology and Parasitology, University of the Andes, Bogotá, Colombia; Dr M. Levin, Institute for Research on Genetic Engineering and Molecular Biology, Buenos Aires, Argentina; Dr M. Postam, "Dr Mario Fatala Chaben" Institute, Buenos Aires, Argentina; Dr A. Rassi, São Salvador Hospital, Goiania, Brazil; Dr J. Marcondes de Rezende, Federal University of Goiás, Goiania, Brazil; Dr A. Rojas de Arias, Institute for Research in Health Sciences, National University of Asunción, Asunción, Paraguay; Dr R. Rosa, Ministry of Health, Montevideo, Uruguay; Dr H. Schenone, Department of Microbiology and Parasitology, University of Chile, Santiago, Chile; Dr E. Segura and Dr D. Solomon, National Centre for the Diagnosis and Study of Endemic Diseases and Epidemics, ANLIS "Dr Carlos G. Malbran", Buenos Aires, Argentina; Dr R. Sica, Ramos Mejía Hospital, Buenos Aires, Argentina; Dr L. Sterin-Borda, School of Medicine and Dentistry, University of Buenos Aires, Argentina; Dr R. Tarleton, Department of Cellular Biology, University of Georgia, Athens, GA, USA; Dr J. Urbina, Biochemical Laboratory, Venezuelan Institute for Scientific Research, Caracas, Venezuela; Dr E. Zerba, Centre for Research on Epidemics and Insecticides, Buenos Aires, Argentina; Dr F. Zicker, Research Capability Strengthening, WHO, Geneva, Switzerland.

References

1. **Laranja FS et al.** Chagas disease. A clinical, epidemiologic and pathologic study. *Circulation*, 1956, **14**:1035–1060.

2. **Rassi A, Rassi A Jr, Rassi GA.** Fase aguda. [Acute phase.] In: Brener Z, Andrade ZA, Barral-Netto M, eds. *Trypanosoma cruzi e doença de Chagas*, 2a ed. [*Trypanosoma cruzi and Chagas disease*, 2nd ed.] Rio de Janeiro, Guanabara Koogan, 2000:231–245.

3. **De Rezende JM, Moreira H.** Forma digestiva da doença de Chagas. [The digestive form of Chagas disease]. In: Brener Z, Andrade ZA, Barral-Netto M, eds. *Trypanosoma cruzi e doença de Chagas*, 2a ed. [*Trypanosoma cruzi and Chagas disease*, 2nd ed.] Rio de Janeiro, Guanabara Koogan, 2000:297–343.

4. **Rosenbaum MB.** Chagasic cardiomyopathy. *Progress in Cardiovascular Disease*, 1964, **3**.199–224.

5. **Sica REP et al.** Involvement of the peripheral sensory nervous system in human chronic Chagas disease. *Medicina*, 1986, **46**:662–668.

6. **De Rezende JM, Luquetti AO.** Chagasic megavisceras. In: *Chagas' disease and the nervous system*. Washington, DC, Pan American Health Organization, 1994:149–171 (Scientific Publication No. 547).

7. **Muñoz P et al.** Enfermedad de Chagas congénita sintomática en recién nacidos y lactantes. [Congenital symptomatic Chagas disease in neonates and breastfed babies.] *Revista Chilena de Pediatría*, 1992, **65**:196–202.

8. **Ferreira MS.** Chagas disease and immunosuppression. *Memorias do Instituto Oswaldo Cruz*, 1999, **97**(Suppl. 1):325–327.

9. **Bocchi EA et al.** Heart transplantation for chronic Chagas heart disease. *Annals of Thoracic Surgery*, 1996, **61**:1727–1733.

10. **Altclas J et al.** Reactivation of chronic Chagas disease following allogenic bone marrow transplantation and successful pre-emptive therapy with benznidazole. *Transplant and Infectious Disease*, 1999, **1**:135–137.

11. **Andrade ZA.** Patologia da doença de Chagas. [Pathology of Chagas disease.] In: Brener Z, Andrade ZA, Barral-Netto M, eds. *Trypanosoma cruzi e doença de Chagas*, 2a ed. [*Trypanosoma cruzi and Chagas disease*, 2nd ed.] Rio de Janeiro, Guanabara Koogan, 2000:201–230.

12. **Higuchi MD et al.** Association of an increase in CD8+ T cells with the presence of *Trypanosoma cruzi* antigens in chronic, human, chagasic myocarditis. *American Journal of Tropical Medicine and Hygiene*, 1997, **56**:485–489.

13. **Tostes S Jr et al.** Miocardite crónica humana: estudo quantivivo dos linfócitos CD4+ e dos CD8+ no exsudato inflamatório. [Chronic human chagasic myocarditis: quantitative study of CD4+ and CD8+ lymphocytes in the inflammatory exudate.] *Revista da Sociedade Brasiliera de Medicina Tropical*, 1994, **27**:127–134.

14. **Reis DA et al.** Characterization of inflammatory infiltrates in chronic chagasic myocardial lesions: presence of tumor necrosis factor-α+ cells and dominance of granzyme A+, CD8+ lymphocytes. *American Journal of Tropical Medicine and Hygiene*, 1993, **48**:637–644.

15. **Lopes MF et al.** Activation-induced CD4+ T cell death by apoptosis in experimental Chagas' disease. *Journal of Immunology*, 1995, **154**:744–752.

16. **Anez N et al.** Myocardial parasite persistence in chronic chagasic patients. *American Journal of Tropical Medicine and Hygiene*, 1999, **60**:726–732.

17. **Vago AR et al.** Genetic characterization of *T. cruzi* directly from tissues of patients with chronic Chagas' disease. Differential distribution of genetic types into diverse organs. *American Journal of Pathology*, 2000, **156**:1805–1809.

18. **Jones EM et al.** Amplification of a *Trypanosoma cruzi* DNA sequence from inflammatory lesions in human chagasic cardiomyopathy. *American Journal of Tropical Medicine and Hygiene*, 1993, **48**:348–357.

19. **Vago AR.** PCR detection of *Trypanosoma cruzi* DNA in oesophageal tissues of patients with chronic digestive Chagas' disease. *Lancet*, 1996, **348**:891.

20. **Rocha A et al.** Pathology of patients with Chagas' disease and acquired immunodeficiency syndrom. *American Journal of Tropical Medicine and Hygiene*, 1994, **50**:261–268.

21. **Kierszenbaum F.** Chagas' disease and the autoimmunity hypothesis. *Clinical Microbiology Reviews*, 1999, **12**:210–223.

22. **Kaplan D et al.** Antibodies to ribosomal P proteins of *Trypanosoma cruzi* in Chagas disease possess functional autoreactivity with heart tissue and differ from anti-P autoantibodies in lupus. *Proceedings of the National Academy of Sciences of the United States of America*, 1997, **94**:10301–10306.

23. **Cunha-Neto E et al.** Autoimmunity in Chagas disease cardiopathy: biological relevance of a cardiac myosin-specific epitope crossreactive to an immunodominant *Trypanosoma cruzi* antigen. *Proceedings of the*

National Academy of Sciences of the United States of America, 1995, **92**:3541–3545.

24. **Goin JC et al.** Functional implication of circulating muscarinic cholinergic receptor autoantibodies in chagasic patients with achalasia. *Gastroenterology*, 1999, **117**:798–805.

25. **Sterin-Borda L, Gorelik G, Borda ES.** Chagasic IgG binding with cardiac muscarinic cholinergic receptors modifies cholinergic-mediated cellular transmembrane signals. *Clinical Immunology and Immunopathology*, 1991, **61**:387–397.

26. **Goin JC et al.** Identification of antibodies with muscarinic cholinergic activity in human Chagas' disease: pathological implications. *Journal of the Autonomic Nervous System*, 1994, **47**:45–52.

27. **Higuchi ML et al.** Immunohistochemical characterization of infiltrating cells in human chronic chagasic myocarditis: comparison with myocardial rejection process. *Virchow Archives of Anatomical Pathology*, 1993, **423**:157–160.

28. **Sztein M, Cuna WR, Kierszenbaum F.** *Trypanosoma cruzi* inhibits the expression of CD3, CD4, CD8 and IL-2R by mitogen-activated helper and cytotoxic human lymphocytes. *Journal of Immunology*, 1990, **144**:3558–3562.

29. **Wincker P et al.** Use of a simplified polymerase chain reaction procedure to detect *Trypanosoma cruzi* in blood samples from chronic patients in rural endemic areas. *American Journal of Tropical Medicine and Hygiene*, 1999, **51**:771–777.

30. **Russomando G et al.** Treatment of congenital Chagas's disease diagnosed and followed up by the polymerase chain reaction. *American Journal of Tropical Medicine and Hygiene*, 1998, **59**:487–491.

31. **Luquetti AO, Rassi A.** Diagnóstico laboratorial da infecçao pelo *Trypanosoma cruzi*. [Laboratory diagnosis of infection by *Trypanosoma cruzi*.] In: Brener Z, Andrade ZA, Barral-Netto M, eds. *Trypanosoma cruzi e doença de Chagas*, 2a ed. [*Trypanosoma cruzi and Chagas disease*, 2nd ed.] Rio de Janeiro, Guanabara Koogan, 2000:344–378.

32. **Moncayo A, Luquetti AO.** Multicentric double blind study for evaluation of *Trypanosoma cruzi* defined antigens as diagnostic reagents. *Memorias do Instituto Oswaldo Cruz*, 1990, **85**:489–495.

33. **Levin MJ et al.** Recombinant *Trypanosoma cruzi* antigens and Chagas' disease diagnosis: analysis of a workshop. *FEMS Microbiology and Immunology*, 1991, **89**:11–20.

34. **Umezawa ES et al.** Evaluation of recombinant antigens for Chagas disease serodiagnosis in South and Central America. *Journal of Clinical Microbiology*, 1999, **37**:1554–1560.

35. **Andrade AL et al.** Randomized trial of efficacy of benznidazole in treatment of early *Trypanosoma cruzi* infection. *Lancet*, 1996, **348**:1407–1413.

36. **Sosa Estani S et al.** Chemotherapy of chronic Chagas' disease with benznidazole in children in the indeterminate phase of Chagas disease. *American Journal of Tropical Medicine and Hygiene*, 1998, **59**:526–529.

37. **Biotti RC et al.** Treatment of chronic Chagas' disease with benznidazole: clinical and serologic evolution of patients with long-term follow-up. *American Heart Journal*, 1994, **127**:151–162.

38. *Tratamiento etiológico de la enfermedad de Chagas. Conclusiones de una Consulta Técnica. [Etiological treatment of Chagas disease. Conclusions of a Technical Consultation.]* Washington, DC, Pan American Health Organization, 1999 (document OPS/HCP/HCT/140/99; available on request from Communicable Dieases, Pan American Health Organization, Washington, DC 20037, USA).

39. **Gutteridge WE.** Designer drugs: pipe-dreams or realities? *Parasitology*, 1997, **114**(Suppl.):S145–S151.

40. **Liendo A, Lazardi K, Urbina JA.** In vitro antiproliferative effects and mechanisms of action of the bis-triazole D0870 and its S(–) enantiomer against *Trypanosoma cruzi*. *Journal of Antimicrobial Chemotherapy*, 1998, **41**:197–205.

41. **Urbina JA.** Chemotherapy of Chagas' disease: the how and the why. *Journal of Molecular Medicine*, 1999, **77**:332–338.

42. **Urbina JA et al.** Antiproliferative effects and mechanism of action of SCH 56592 against *Trypanosoma (Schizotrypanum) cruzi*: in vitro and in vivo studies. *Antimicrobial Agents and Chemotherapy*, 1998, **42**:1771–1777.

43. **Andrade SG.** Caracterização de cepas do *Trypanosoma cruzi* isoladas do Recôncavo Baiano. [Characterization of strains of *Trypanosoma cruzi* found in the Recôncavo Baiano.] *Revista de Patologia Tropical*, 1974, **3**:65–121.

44. **Miles MA et al.** Further enzymic characters of *Trypanosoma cruzi* and their evaluation for strain identification. *Transactions of the Royal Society of Tropical Medicine and Hygiene*, 1980, **74**:221–242.

45. **Tibayrenc M.** Population genetics of parasitic protozoa and other microorganisms. *Advances in Parasitology*, 1995, **36**:48–115.

46. **Morel CM et al.** Strains and clones of *Trypanosoma cruzi* can be characterized by restriction endonuclease fingerprinting of kinetoplast DNA minicircles. *Proceedings of the National Academy of Sciences of the United States of America*, 1980, **77**:6810–6814.

47. **Souto RP et al.** DNA markers define two major phylogenetic lineages of *Trypanosoma cruzi*. *Molecular Biochemistry and Parasitology*, 1996, **83**:141–152.

48. **Zingales B et al.** Molecular epidemiology of American trypanosomiasis in Brazil based on dimorphisms of rRNA and mini-exon gene sequences. *International Journal of Parasitology*, 1998, **28**:105–112.

49. Recommendations from a satellite meeting. *Memorias do Instituto Oswaldo Cruz*, 1999, **94**(Suppl. 1):429–432.

50. **Clark CG, Pung OJ.** Host specificity of ribosomal DNA variants in sylvatic *Trypanosoma cruzi* from North America. *Molecular and Biochemical Parasitology*, 1994, **66**:175–179.

51. **Romanha AJ et al.** Isoenzyme patterns of cultured *Trypanosoma cruzi*: changes after prolonged subculture. *Comparative Biochemical Physiology*, 1979, **62B**:139–142.

52. **Fernandes O et al.** Brazilian isolates of *Trypanosoma cruzi* from humans and triatomines classified into two lineages using mini-exon and ribosomal RNA sequences. *American Journal of Tropical Medicine and Hygiene*, 1998, **58**:807–811.

53. **Brenière SF et al.** Different behaviour of two *Trypanosoma cruzi* major clones: transmission and circulation in young Bolivian patients. *Experimental Parasitology*, 1998, **89**:285–295.

54. **Zingales B et al.** *Trypanosoma cruzi* genome project: biological characteristics and molecular typing of clone CL Brener. *Acta Tropica*, 1997, **68**:159–173.

55. **Hanke J et al.** Hybridization mapping of *Trypanosoma cruzi* chromosomes III and IV. *Electrophoresis*, 1998, **4**:482–485.

56. **Henriksson J et al.** Chromosome specific markers reveal conserved linkage groups in spite of extensive chromosomal size variation in *Trypanosoma cruzi*. *Molecular Biochemistry and Parasitology*, 1995, **73**:63–74.

57. **Di Noia JM et al.** The *Trypanosoma cruzi* mucin family is transcribed from hundreds of genes having hypervariable regions. *Journal of Biological Chemistry*, 1998, **273**:10843–10850.

58. **Lent H et al.** Addenda et corrigenda. In: Carcavallo RU et al., eds. *Atlas of Chagas' disease vectors in the Americas. Vol. 3*. Rio de Janeiro, FIOCRUZ, 1999:1183–1192.

59. **Carcavallo RU et al.** Geographical distribution and alti-latitudinal dispersion. In: Carcavallo RU et al., eds. *Atlas of Chagas'disease vectors in the Americas. Vol. 3*. Rio de Janeiro, FIOCRUZ, 1999:747–792.

60. **Curto de Casas SI et al.** Bioclimatic factors and zones of life. In: Carcavallo RU et al., eds. *Atlas of Chagas' disease vectors in the Americas. Vol. 3*. Rio de Janeiro, FIOCRUZ, 1999:793–838.

61. **Pereira H et al.** Comparative kinetics of bloodmeal intake by *Triatoma infestans* and *Rhodnius prolixus*, the two principal vectors of Chagas disease. *Medical and Veterinary Entomology*, 1998, **12**:84–88.

62. **Silveira AC.** Current status of vector transmission control of Chagas' disease in the Americas. In: Carcavallo RU et al., eds. *Atlas of Chagas' disease vectors in the Americas. Vol. 3*. Rio de Janeiro, FIOCRUZ, 1999:1160–1182.

63. **Lopez G, Moreno J.** Genetic variability and differentiation between populations of *Rhodnius prolixus* and *R. pallescens*, vectors of Chagas disease in Colombia. *Memorias do Instituto Oswaldo Cruz*, 1995, **90**:353–357.

64. **Casini CE et al.** Morphometric differentiation evidenced between two geographic populations of *Triatoma infestans* in Paraguay. *Research and Reviews in Parasitology*, 1995, **55**:25–30.

65. **Dujardin JP et al.** Uso de marcadores genéticos en la vigilancia entomologica de la enfermedad de Chagas. [Use of genetic markers in entomological surveillance of Chagas disease.] In: Cassab JA, Noireau F, Guillen G, eds. *La enfermedad de Chagas en Bolivia — conociemientos científicos al inicio del programa de control (1998–2002). [Chagas disease in Bolivia — scientific knowledge at the start of the control programme (1998–2002).]* La Paz, Ministry of Health and Social Welfare: 157–169.

66. **Dujardin JP, Bermudez H, Schofield CJ.** The use of morphometrics in entomological surveillance of sylvatic foci of *Triatoma infestans* in Bolivia. *Acta Tropica*, 1997, **66**:145–153.

67. **Dujardin JP, Schofield CJ, Tibayrenc M.** Population structure of Andean *Triatoma infestans*: allozyme frequencies and their epidemiological relevance. *Medical and Veterinary Entomology*, 1998, **12**:20–29.

68. **Dias JCP.** Epidemiología. [Epidemiology.] In: Brener Z, Andrade ZA, Barral-Netto M, eds. *Trypanosoma cruzi e doença de Chagas*, 2a ed. [*Trypanosoma cruzi and Chagas disease*, 2nd ed.] Rio de Janeiro, Guanabara-Koogan, 2000:55–58.

69. **Wisnivesky-Colli C et al.** Epidemiological role of humans, dogs and cats in the transmission of *Trypanosoma cruzi* in a central area of Argentina. *Revista do Instituto de Medicina Tropical de São Paulo*, 1985, **27**:346–352.

70. **Gürtler RE et al.** Dynamics of transmission of *Trypanosoma cruzi* in a rural area of Argentina. I. The dog reservoir: an epidemiological profile. *Revista do Instituto de Medicina Tropical de São Paulo*, 1986, **28**:28–35.

71. **Schweigmann NJ et al.** Estudio de la prevalencia de la infección por *Trypanosoma cruzi* en zarigüeyas (*Didelphis albiventris*) en Santiago del Estero, Argentina. [Study of the prevalence of *Trypanosoma cruzi* in opossum (*Didelphis albiventris*) in Santiago del Estero, Argentina.] *Pan American Journal of Public Health*, 1999, **6**:371–377.

72. **Moncayo A.** Progress towards interruption of transmission of Chagas disease. *Memorias do Instituto Oswaldo Cruz*, 1999, **94**(Suppl. 1):401–404.

73. **Schmunis G, Zicker F, Moncayo A.** Interruption of Chagas' disease transmission through vector elimination. *Lancet*, 1997, **348**:1171.

74. **Segura EL et al.** Decrease in the prevalence of infection by *Trypanosoma cruzi* (Chagas' disease) in young men of Argentina. *Bulletin of the Pan American Health Organization*, 1985, **19**:252–264.

75. *Reports of the Intergovernmental Commission of the Southern Cone Initiative.* Washington, DC, Pan American Health Organization, 1998–1999.

76. **Camargo M et al.** Inquérito sorológico de la prevalência de la infecção chagasica no Brasil, 1975–1980. [Serological survey of the prevalence of Chagas' infection in Brazil, 1975–1980.] *Revista do Instituto de Medicina Tropical de São Paulo*, 1984, **26**:192–204.

77. Chagas disease: interruption of transmission in Brazil. *Weekly Epidemiological Record*, 2000, **75**:153–155.

78. **Schenone H et al.** Enfermedad de Chagas en Chile. Sectores rurales y periurbanos del area endemoenzootica. Relación entre las condiciones habitacionales, infestación triatominica domiciliar e infección por *Trypanosoma cruzi* en el vector, humanos y animales domésticos. [Chagas' disease in Chile. Rural and periurban sectors of the endemo-enzootic area. Relationship between housing conditions, domiciliary triatomid infestation and infection by *Trypanosoma cruzi* of the vector, humans and domestic animals.] *Boletín Chileno de Parasitología*, 1985, **40**:58–67.

79. Chagas disease: interruption of transmission in Chile. *Weekly Epidemiological Record*, 2000, **75**:10–12.

80. **Cerisola JA et al.** Chagas disease and blood transfusion. *Boletín de la Oficina Sanitaria Panamericana*, 1972, **73**:203–221.

81. **Salvatella R et al.** Seroprevalencia de anticuerpos contra *Trypanosoma cruzi* en 13 departamentos del Uruguay. [Seroprevalence of antibodies against *Trypanosoma cruzi* in 13 departments of Uruguay.] *Boletín de la Oficina Sanitaria Panamericana*, 1989:108–117.

82. Chagas disease: interruption of transmission in Uruguay. *Weekly Epidemiological Record*, 1998, **73**:1–4.

83. **Alzogaray R, Zerba E.** Evaluation of hyperactivity produced by pyrethroid treatment on third instar nymphs of *Triatoma infestans*. *Archives of Insect Biochemistry and Physiology*, 1997, **35**:323–333.

84. OMS protocolo de evaluación de efecto insecticida sobre tríatominos [WHO protocol for the evaluation of insecticidal effect on triatomines.] *Acta Toxicológica Argentina*, 1994, **2**:29–32.

85. **Vassena CV, Picollo MI, Zerba EN.** Insecticide resistance in Brazilian *Triatoma infestans* and Venezuelan *Rhodnius prolixus*. *Medical and Veterinary Entomology*, 2000, **14**:1–5.

86. **Silveira AC, Vinhaes M.** Elimination of vector-borne transmission of Chagas disease. *Memorias do Instituto Oswaldo Cruz*, 1999, **94**(Suppl. 1):405–411.

87. **Salvatella R et al.** Seroprevalencia de la infección por *Trypanosoma cruzi* en escolares de 6 y 12 años de edad de tres departamentos endémicos de Uruguay. [Seroprevalence of infection by *Trypanosoma cruzi* in 6- and 12-year-old schoolchildren in three endemic departments of Uruguay.] *Boletín Chileno de Parasitología*, 1999, **54**:51–56.

88. **Lorca M et al.** Evaluación de los programas de erradicación de la enfermedad de Chagas en Chile mediante estudio serológico de niños menores de 10 años. [Evaluation of programmes for the eradication of Chagas disease in Chile by the serological study of children less than 10 years old.] *Boletín Chileno de Parasitología*, 1996, **51**:80–85.

89. World Bank. *World development report 1993: investing in health.* Oxford, Oxford University Press, 1993:216–218.

90. *The World Health Report 2000. Health systems: improving performance.* Geneva, World Health Organization, 2000.

91. **Akhavan D.** *Analysis of cost-effectiveness of the Chagas disease control programme.* Brasilia, Ministry of Health, National Health Foundation, 1997.

92. *Chagas disease: progress towards interruption of transmission in Venezuela. Weekly Epidemiological Record*, 1999, **74**:289–296.

93. **Ponce C.** Elimination of the vectorial transmission of Chagas disease in Central American countries. *Memorias do Instituto Oswaldo Cruz*, 1999, **94**(Suppl. 1):417–418.

Annex 1
Safety precautions for laboratory work with
Trypanosoma cruzi

All personnel handling either *Trypanosoma cruzi*, in vitro or in vivo, or infected triatomines must, first, be expert in general laboratory procedures, second, know the techniques specially related to *T. cruzi*, and third, have a good background knowledge of the parasite. Initially they must also work under close supervision. The following must be considered as additional precautions essential to the safety of competent research workers and their technicians:

1. Access to the laboratory, animal rooms, and insectary must be limited to those people actually working on the organism, and these areas must be clearly marked.
2. Secure barriers must be provided to prevent the escape of infected animals or insects.
3. A suitable protocol must be provided on the methods to be used for the disposal of dead infected animals and insects (e.g. autoclaving or incineration).
4. The following protective clothing must be worn:
   — face mask
   — back-fastening gown
   — gloves
   — shoes (not sandals).
5. Nothing must be pipetted by mouth.
6. The apparatus and procedures must be designed to reduce hazards (e.g. safety boxes for homogenizers, caps for centrifuge tubes, and safety hoods for subculturing must be provided).
7. A suitable protocol must be provided for the decontamination of glassware, etc. (e.g. disinfectant autoclaving).
8. Maintenance staff, the fire service, etc., must be informed of the nature of the work being carried out.
9. The medical staff of the organization must be informed of the nature of the work being carried out so that suitable procedures can be established for the monitoring of accidents and the treatment of the personnel involved.
10. All staff must be monitored periodically (e.g. every 6 months) for *T. cruzi* antibodies.
11. A protocol to be followed in the event of a suspected accident must be provided, as follows:
    (a) Clean the skin immediately with ethanol or a disinfectant.
    (b) Report the accident to the appropriate medical person.

(c) If there is only a slight risk of infection, monitor blood for the next few months.

(d) If the risk of infection is high, treat with nifurtimox or benznidazole.

(e) Report the accident, if required, to the public health authority.

12. All staff must be given a copy of the accident protocol and they must be properly instructed in how to carry it out. It is important that they should be aware of possible dangers so that they will avoid a casual approach. It is equally important that they should not be frightened of working with the organism.

Recommendation. When a confirmed accident does occur, treatment with benznidazole should be started immediately and continued for 10 days without waiting for evidence of infection.

Annex 2
Labelling of *Trypanosoma cruzi* isolates

In accordance with the recommendations of a meeting (Panama, 1985) organized by the UNDP/World Bank/WHO Special Programme for Research and Training in Tropical Diseases on standardization of methods for *T. cruzi* classification,[1] the code for the designation of isolates should consist of four elements, separated by oblique strokes:

1. *The type of host animal or vector from which the strain was isolated.* A four-letter code should be used, the first indicating the class to which the animal or vector belongs (M for Mammalia, I for Insecta) followed by three letters indicating the generic name of the host or "000" if the host has not yet been identified. Table A2.1 gives the code letters to be used for mammalian genera.
2. *The country in which the isolation was made.* The country of isolation is indicated by the two-letter codes shown in Table A2.2.
3. *The year of isolation.* This is indicated by the last two digits or "00" if unknown.
4. *The laboratory designation* (e.g. laboratory code and serial number).

Standard reference strains of *T. cruzi* are listed in Table A2.3.

---

[1] *Report of a meeting on the standardization of methods for* Trypanosoma cruzi *classification.* Geneva, World Health Organization, 1985 (unpublished document TDR/EPICHA-TCC/85.3; available on request from UNDP/World Bank/WHO Special Programme for Research and Training in Tropical Diseases, World Health Organization, 1211 Geneva 27, Switzerland).

Table A2.1

Generic codes for labelling _T. cruzi_ isolates from mammals[a] according to the proposed international code

AKO	_Akodon_ (ROD)		LAS	_Lasiurus_ (CHT)
ALO	_Alouatta_ (PMT)		LUT	_Lutreolina_ (MSP)
ANO	_Anoura_ (CHT)		MAR	_Marmosa_ (MSP)
AOT	_Aotus_ (PMT)		MEP	_Mephitis_ (CAR)
ART	_Artibeus_ (CHT)		MET	_Metachirus_ (MSP)
ATE	_Ateles_ (PMT)		MIM	_Mimon_ (CHT)
BAS	_Bassaricyon_ (CAR)		MIN	_Micronycteris_ (CHT)
BRA	_Bradypus_ (EDE)		MOL	_Molossops_ (CHT)
CAA	_Capra_ (ARD)		MON	_Monodelphis_ (MSP)
CAB	_Cabassous_ (EDE)		MOR	_Mormoops_ (CHT)
CAI	_Carollia_ (CHT)		MOS	_Molossus_ (CHT)
CAL	_Caluromys_ (MSP)		MUS	_Mus_ (ROD)
CAN	_Canis_ (CAR)		MYO	_Myotis_ (CHT)
CAO	_Calomys_ (ROD)		NAS	_Nasua_ (CAR)
CAV	_Cavia_ (ROD)		NEC	_Nectomys_ (ROD)
CBL	_Cebuella_ (PMT)		NEO	_Neotoma_ (ROD)
CEB	_Cebus_ (PMT)		NOC	_Noctilio_ (CHT)
CEM	_Cercomys_ (ROD)		OCT	_Octodon_ (ROD)
CER	_Cerdocyon_ (CAR)		ORT	_Oryctolagus_ (LGM)
CHO	_Choloepus_ (EDE)		ORY	_Oryzomys_ (ROD)
CHP	_Chaetophractus_ (EDE)		OXY	_Oxymycterus_ (ROD)
CIT	_Citellus_ (ROD)		PER	_Peromyscus_ (ROD)
CLC	_Callicebus_ (PMT)		PET	_Peroteryx_ (CHT)
CLX	_Callithrix_ (PMT)		PHI	_Philander_ (MSP)
COE	_Coendou_ (ROD)		PHS	_Phyllostomus_ (CHT)
CON	_Conepatus_ (CAR)		PHT	_Phyllotis_ (ROD)
CUN	_Cuniculus_ (ROD)		POT	_Potos_ (CAR)
DAP	_Dasyprocta_ (ROD)		PRC	_Procyon_ (CAR)
DAS	_Dasypus_ (ROD)		PRO	_Proechimys_ (ROD)
DES	_Desmodus_ (CHT)		RAT	_Rattus_ (ROD)
DIA	_Diaemus_ (CHT)		RHN	_Rhynophylla_ (CHT)
DID	_Didelphis_ (MSP)		RHT	_Rhynchonycteris_ (CHT)
DPM	_Diplomys_ (ROD)		SAC	_Saccopteryx_ (CHT)
DUS	_Dusicyon_ (CAR)		SAG	_Saguinus_ (PMT)
ECH	_Echimys_ (ROD)		SAI	_Saimiri_ (PMT)
EIR	_Eira_ (CAR)		SCI	_Sciurus_ (ROD)
EPT	_Eptesicus_ (CHT)		SIG	_Sigmodon_ (ROD)
EUM	_Eumops_ (CHT)		STU	_Sturnira_ (CHT)
EUP	_Euphractus_ (EDE)		SUS	_Sus_ (ARD)
FEL	_Felis_ (CAR)		SYL	_Sylvilagus_ (LGM)
GAL	_Galea_ (ROD)		TAD	_Tadarida_ (CHT)
GAT	_Galictis_ (CAR)		TAM	_Tamandua_ (EDE)
GLO	_Glossophaga_ (CHT)		THO	_Thomasomys_ (ROD)
HET	_Heteromys_ (ROD)		TOL	_Tolypeutes_ (EDE)
HIS	_Histiotus_ (CHT)		TRA	_Trachops_ (CHT)
HOM	_Homo_ (PMT)		TYL	_Tylomys_ (ROD)

Table A2.1 (*continued*)
Generic codes for labelling *T. cruzi* isolates from mammals[a] according to the proposed international code

URD	*Uroderma* (CHT)	VAR	*Vampyrum* (CHT)
URO	*Urocyon* (CAR)	WIE	*Wiedomys* (ROD)
VAM	*Vampyrodes* (CHT)	ZAE	*Zaedyus* (EDE)
VAP	*Vampyrops* (CHT)	ZYG	*Zygodontomys* (ROD)

[a] ARD = Artiodactyla; CAR = Carnivora; CHT = Chiroptera; EDE = Edentata; LGM = Lagomorpha; MSP = Marsupiala; PMT = Primates; ROD = Rodentia.

Table A2.2
Designation of endemic countries or territories according to the codes developed by the International Organization for Standardization (ISO)

Argentina	AR	Guyana	GY
Bahamas	BS	French Guiana	GF
Barbados	BB	Honduras	HN
Brazil	BR	Mexico	MX
Bolivia	BO	Nicaragua	NI
Chile	CL	Panama	PA
Colombia	CO	Paraguay	PY
Costa Rica	CR	Peru	PE
El Salvador	SV	Suriname	SR
Ecuador	EC	Uruguay	UY
Guatemala	GT	Venezuela	VE

Table A2.3
Standard reference strains of *T. cruzi*

MHOM/PE/00/Peru	MHOM/BR/82/Dm-28c[a]
MHOM/BR/00/12-SF	MHOM/BR/78?/Sylvio-X10-CL1[a]
MHOM/CO/00/Colombia	MHOM/BR/78/Sylvio-X10-CL4[a]
MHOM/BR/00/Y	MHOM/BR/77/Esmeraldo-CL3[a]
MHOM/CL/00/Tulahuen	MHOM/BR/68/CAN-III-CL1[a]
MHOM/AR/74/CA-1[a]	MHOM/BR/68/CAN-III-CL2[a]
MHOM/AR/74/CA-1-72[a]	MHOM/BO/80/CNT-92:80-CL1[a]
MHOM/AR/00/CA-1-78[a]	IINF/BO/80/Sc43-CL1[a]
MHOM/AR/00/Miranda-83[a]	IINF/PY/81/P63-CL[a]
MHOM/AR/00/Miranda-88[a]	MHOM/AR/78/RA
	(low virulence strain)

[a] Derived from clonal populations.

The minimal data that should be applied with any isolate sent for identification are:

1. Host
   (i)   Scientific name
   (ii) Clinical form
   (iii) Organ or tissue
2. Geographical origin
   (i)   Country
   (ii) State
   (iii) Locality
   (iv) Map coordinates
3. Date of isolation
   Day/Month/Year
4. Name of laboratory
   Name (and initials) of research worker
5. Laboratory number of isolate
6. Mode of conservation
7. Identification methods used
   (i)   Method(s)
   (ii) Result(s)
8. Other observations

Annex 3
List of sylvatic and domestic or peridomestic animal reservoir hosts of *Trypanosoma cruzi* and countries in which they have been found infected[1,2]

I. Sylvatic Mammals

Order MARSUPIALIA

Family DIDELPHIDAE

Caluromys derbianus, Costa Rica, Panama.

Caluromys lanatus, Brazil (Minas Gerais), Venezuela.

Caluromys philander, French Guiana, Venezuela.

Didelphis albiventris (= *D. paraguayensis*; = *D. azarae*), Argentina, Bolivia, Brazil (Ceará, Minas Gerais, São Paulo, Santa Catarina), Uruguay.

Didelphis marsupialis, Brazil, Colombia, Costa Rica, Ecuador, French Guiana, Guatemala, Honduras, Mexico, Panama, USA, Venezuela.

Lutreolina crassicaudata, Argentina, Brazil (São Paulo).

Marmosa agilis, Brazil.

Marmosa alstoni, Costa Rica.

Marmosa elegans, Argentina, Brazil.

Marmosa microtarsus, Brazil.

Marmosa murina, Colombia.

Marmosa pusilia, Argentina.

Marmosa robinsoni, Venezuela.

Metachirus nudicaudatus, Brazil.

Monodelphis brevicaudata, Venezuela.

Monodelphis domestica, Brazil.

Philander opossum, Brazil, Colombia, Costa Rica, Panama.

Order EDENTATA

Family MYRMECOPHAGIDAE

Tamandua tetradactyla, Brazil, Colombia, Panama, Venezuela.

Family BRADYPODIDAE

Bradypus infuscatus, Colombia, Panama.

Choloepus hoffmanni, Panama.

Family DASYPODIDAE

Cabassous tatouay, Argentina.

Cabassous unicinctus, Argentina, Brazil, French Guiana, Venezuela.

Chaetophractus vellerosus, Argentina.

Chaetophractus villosus, Argentina.

Dasypus kapleri, Colombia, Venezuela.

Dasypus novemcinctus, Argentina, Brazil, Colombia, Costa Rica, French Guiana, Guatemala, Mexico, USA, Venezuela.

Euphractus sexcinctus, Brazil, Venezuela.

Tolypeutes matacus, Argentina.

Zaedyus pichiy, Argentina.

Order CHIROPTERA

Family EMBALLONURIDAE

Peroteryx macrotis, Colombia.

Rhynchonycteris naso, Colombia.

Saccopteryx bilineata, Colombia, Venezuela.

Family NOCTILIONIDAE

Noctilio albiventris, Brazil, Colombia.

Noctilio leporinus, Colombia.

---

[1] For some species *T. cruzi* was not formally identified.
[2] Largely following the systematics for Central and South American mammals of Cabrera A. Catálogo de los mamíferos de America del Sur. *Revista des Museo Argentino de Ciencias Naturales "Bernadino Rivadavia"* ... , 4:1–732 (1957–61); and for North American mammals of Hall ER, Kelson KR. *The mammals of North America*. New York, Ronald, 1959 (rev. 1981 by Hall).

Family PHYLLOSTOMIDAE

Anoura caudifera, Brazil.

Artibeus jamaicensis, Brazil.

Artibeus lituratus, Colombia, French Guiana, Venezuela.

Carollia castanea, Colombia.

Carollia perspicillata, Brazil, Colombia, Panama, Venezuela.

Carollia subrufa, Colombia.

Carollia villosum, Colombia.

Glossophaga soricina, Brazil, Colombia, Panama.

Micronycteris branchyotis, Colombia.

Micronycteris minuta, Colombia.

Mimon bennettii, Colombia.

Mormoops megalophylla, Colombia.

Phyllostomus discolor, Colombia.

Sturnira tildae, Colombia.

Phyllostomus elongatus, Brazil, Venezuela.

Phyllostomus hastatus, Argentina, Colombia, French Guiana, Panama, Venezuela.

Rhinophylla pumilio, Colombia.

Sturnira lilium, Colombia.

Sturnira tildae, Colombia.

Trachops cirrhosus, Brazil.

Uroderma bilobatum, Colombia, Panama

Vampyrodes caraccioloi, Colombia.

Vampyrops helleri, Colombia.

Vampyrum spectrum, Colombia.

Family DESMODONTIDAE

Desmodus rotundus, Brazil, Colombia, Panama, Venezuela.

Diaemus youngi, Colombia.

Family VESPERTILIONIDAE

Eptesicus brasiliensis, Argentina, Brazil.

Eptesicus furinalis, Argentina.

Histiotus montanus, Argentina.

Lasiurus borealis, Argentina.

Lasiurus cinereus, Brazil.

Lasiurus ega, Brazil.

Myotis nigricans, Colombia.

Family MOLOSSIDAE

Eumops auripendulus, Brazil.

Eumops bonariensis, Argentina.

Eumops glaucinus, Brazil.

Eumops perotis, Brazil.

Eumops trumbulli, Colombia.

Molossops temminckii, Colombia.

Molossus bondae, Colombia.

Molossus molossus, Brazil, Colombia, Venezuela.

Tadarida laticaudata, Brazil.

Order CARNIVORA

Family CANIDAE

Cerdocyon thous, Argentina, Brazil.

Dusicyon culpaeus, Argentina, Chile.

Dusicyon griseus, Argentina, Chile.

Dusicyon vetulus, Brazil.

Urocyon cinereoargenteus, USA.

Family PROCYONIDAE

Bassaricyon gabbii, Panama.

Nasua nasua, Argentina, Brazil.

Nasua narica, Belize, Costa Rica, Panama.

Potos flavus, Panama.

Procyon cancrivorus, Brazil, Venezuela.

Procyon lotor, Costa Rica, Guatemala, USA.

Family MUSTELIDAE

Conepatus semistriatus, Costa Rica.

Eira barbara, Argentina, Brazil, Colombia.

Galictis cuja, Argentina, Brazil.

Galictis vittata, Brazil.

Mephitis mephitis, USA.

Family FELIDAE

Felis yaguaroundi, Argentina.

Order LAGOMORPHA

Family LEPORIDAE

Sylvilagus floridanus

Sylvilagus orinoci

Order RODENTIA

Family SCIURIDAE

Citellus leucurus, USA.

Sciurus aestuans, Brazil, Venezuela.

Sciurus granatensis, Panama, Venezuela.
Sciurus ignitus, Argentina.
Sciurus igniventris, Colombia.
Family HETEROMYIDAE
Heteromys anomalus, Venezuela.
Family CRICETIDAE
Akodon arviculoides, Brazil.
Akodon lasiotis, Brazil.
Akodon nigritus, Brazil.
Calomys expulsus, Brazil.
Calomys laucha, Argentina.
Calomys toner, Brazil.
Nectomys squamipes, Brazil.
Neotoma albigula, USA.
Neotoma fuscipes, USA.
Neotoma micropus, USA.
Oryzomys capito, Brazil.
Oryzomys concolor, Venezuela.
Oryzomys nigripes, Brazil.
Oryzomys subflavus, Brazil.
Oxymcterus hispidus, Brazil.
Peromyscus boylii, USA.
Peromyscus truei, USA.
Phyllotis griseoflavus, Argentina.
Sigmodon hispidus, Colombia, El Salvador.
Thomasomys dorsalis, Brazil.
Tylomys panamensis, Panama.
Wiedomys pirrhorhinus, Brazil.
Zygodontomys lasiurus, Brazil.
Family OCTODONTIDAE
Octodon degus, Chile.
Family ECHIMYIDAE
Cercomys cunicularius, Brazil.
Diplomys labilis, Panama.
Echimys semivillosus, Venezuela.
Proechimys guayanensis, Colombia.
Proechimys semispinosus, Panama, Venezuela.
Family CAVIIDAE
Cavia sp., Brazil.
Cavia aperea, Brazil.

Galea spixii, Brazil.
Family DASYPROCTIDAE
Dasyprocta aguti, Brazil, Venezuela.
Dasyprocta azarae, Brazil.
Dasyprocta fuliginosa, Colombia.
Dasyprocta punctata, Ecuador, Panama.
Family AGOUTIDAE
Cuniculus paca, Venezuela.
Family ERETHIZONTIDAE
Coendou insidiosus, Brazil.
Coendou mexicanus, Costa Rica.
Coendou prehensilis, Venezuela.
Coendou rothschildi, Colombia.
Coendou vestitus, Venezuela.

Order PRIMATES
Family CEBIDAE
Alouatta caraya, Brazil.
Alouatta senicula, Colombia, Venezuela.
Aotus trivirgatus, Panama.
Ateles belzebuth, Colombia.
Ateles fuscipes, Panama.
Ateles geoffroyi, Colombia.
Callicebus nigrifrons, Brazil.
Callicebus ornatus, Colombia.
Cebus albifrons, Colombia.
Cebus apella, Brazil, Colombia, French Guiana, Venezuela.
Cebus capucinus, Colombia, Panama, Venezuela.
Saimiri oerstedii, Panama.
Saimiri sciureus, Brazil, Colombia, Panama, Peru.
Family CALLITHRICIDAE
Callithrix argentata, Brazil.
Callithrix geoffroyi, Brazil.
Callithrix jacchus, Brazil.
Callithrix penicillata, Brazil.
Cebuella pygmaea, Colombia.
Saguinus geoffroyi, Panama.
Saguinus leucopus, Colombia.
Saguinus nigricollis, Colombia.

II. Domestic and Peridomestic Mammals

Canis familiaris

Capra hyrcus

Cavia porcellus

Felis domesticus

Mus musculus

Oryctolagus cuniculus

Rattus norvegicus

Rattus rattus

Sus scrofa